69 Sex P

69 Sex Positions for
69 Nights of Pleasure

A Practical Sex Guide

Olivia Love

Contents

Introduction

We all think about sex. It's ok. Don't deny it! On average, men think about sex about 19 times a day, and women have 10 sexual thoughts a day. Sex is a part of who we are. However, we spend a lot more time thinking about it rather than doing something with those thoughts.

With this book, you've taken a substantial first step in adding variety to your sex life, and as we all know, variety is the spice of life! It is more so when it comes to sex. Patterns, comfort zones, and routines plague many couples in the bedroom. Kudos to you for being brave enough to push your boundaries and open your mind! You will not regret it.

The following 69 positions offer you guidance as you embark on a new sexual adventure. There are detailed descriptions of every posture covering the basic positions and variations to try. Frank discussions about intimacy and sexual health accompany the positions as well as some general tips for giving and receiving pleasure.

This guide will give you the basics and hopefully enough confidence to experiment on your own. Good luck on your sexual journey to a more balanced state of sexual health, a more intimate relationship with your partner, and the best sex you've ever had!

Intimacy

Sex is a physical expression of intimacy. It often embodies deep feelings and connections, but this isn't a foregone conclusion. The act of sex can be strictly physical with little or no real intimacy between partners. However, the physical act itself will inevitably build some level of intimacy especially if it is a recurrent event. Just physically sharing a sexual encounter will not create a well-balanced, deep, intimate connection that many people seek with their partners, but intimacy requires more than just physical contact. Intimacy in sex can increase pleasure, build stronger bonds between partners, and offer a way to express feelings and emotions that can sometimes be hard to put into words.

Intimacy is the key to having good sex. None of the positions in this book will offer you greater pleasure than being truly intimate with your partner. To achieve intimacy, there are a couple of things that need to be in place. First, you must allow yourself to open to giving and receiving pleasure. You must believe that you are entitled to and need the pleasure that you are getting as well as offering it to your partner. This can be difficult, and it requires an open heart, mind, and attitude to the experience and your partner. Intimacy is often viewed as scary because of the level of vulnerability it demands from people. Trust yourself, trust your partner, and together the two of you can become something greater than the sum of your parts.

A few tips on how to go about this tricky business of intimacy:

Eyes wide open: It is hard to connect with someone who won't look at you. Eye contact is a way of connecting with people. You make eye contact with people all day long. Don't overlook this simple, yet critical, step in building an intimate connection. Look into your lover's eyes and let them see into yours. You'd be surprised what can be communicated without any words at all.

Don't forget the foreplay: Foreplay is essential to intimacy. During the act of sex, the nuances of your partner's reactions and desires can be lost in the pleasure or intensity of the moment. Foreplay allows for exploration, connection, and arousal and should not be rushed or skipped.

Light it up: Sex in the dark feels safe, and people sometimes find themselves able to relax more if the cloak of darkness is pulled tightly around them. However, darkness is a barrier to intimacy. Turn on the lights, and let your partner see you (and vice versa!). It needn't be a beacon or a spotlight; a simple candle or a nightlight is a good place to start.

Scary at first, it can help you be more comfortable in your relationship as well as your own skin!

Don't be afraid to laugh: Few people are capable of pulling off a movie production sex session. We get a cramp, lose our balance, or make a funny noise. Laughter in the bedroom is not something that should be taboo. It is ok to laugh at things that don't go right. It lightens the mood and creates a safe place for when things do not go as planned. A safe, non-judgemental environment will set the stage for experimentation and open communication.

Intimacy requires effort and time, but it is well worth it in the end. It will take your relationship to a new level and open the door for amazing sex.

Sexual Health

The concept of sexual health is far broader than most people realize. Most narrow definitions include the protection from disease and the prevention of unwanted pregnancy. However, it goes far beyond this. Sexual health includes being educated about sex, dealing with sexual dysfunctions, maintaining healthy attitudes about sex, and being able to participate in pleasurable, consensual, safe sex.

That's a lot to take in, but let's start with the basics. Obviously, if you are sexually active, you must be responsible. You must be open and honest with your partner about any sexual diseases or issues you may have, and they should reciprocate. If your partner is not willing to participate in a full disclosure of their sexual health, you probably should rethink your relationship. You should take necessary precautions including protection like condoms and birth control. These are common sense but are of paramount importance. Without covering these bases, the ramifications of having sex could wreck your sexual health in life-altering ways.

Moving past the basics, consider the attitudes and stigmas that exist around sex. How do your attitudes and beliefs impact your sexual health? A healthy attitude toward sex includes the openness to discuss it with your partner, a desire to experience and give pleasure, and the ability to distinguish between your feelings and societal bias. Only with an open mind can you obtain optimal sexual health.

Increasing your knowledge base is another crucial facet of maintaining good sexual health. The Internet can be a scary place to look around for sexual health information and to avoid being inundated by porn or sex ads. However, there are many credible websites with excellent information on how you can improve your sexual health. Your physician should also be a good resource for any questions you may have. Whatever your resource, expanding your knowledge on the topic of sex can only illuminate you and improve your overall sexual well-being.

Sexual dysfunction is an uncomfortable topic for most people to consider. Issues that prevent you from enjoying sex are important and shouldn't be ignored just because they are difficult to talk about. You wouldn't hesitate to go to the doctor if your hand stopped working. Your sexual function is no less critical to your overall good health. Frustrations in the bedroom will manifest in other areas of your life so do not ignore these issues. Talk to a medical provider if something isn't right. Don't forget to talk to your partner as well. While this conversation is as appealing as root canal treatment, it is vital to maintain open, honest communication about sex and any issues you or your partner are having.

Sexual health is an often overlooked part of overall health. Just like maintaining a healthy weight and getting regular exercise, sex is an essential aspect of your physical body that shouldn't be forgotten. Embrace your sexual self. Nurture that aspect of yourself as intentionally as you eat your fruits and vegetables. Balanced sexual health will augment other healthy habits and lead you to better health, happier relationships, and of course, more pleasurable sex!

Positions

Experimenting with positions is a great way to spice up your sex life. Keep an open mind, and don't be afraid to push your limits! There are so many more ways to enjoy sex beyond the typical trio- missionary, doggie, and cowgirl. Leave your ideas of movie sex at the door. It doesn't have to look a certain way or be exactly as described. Make it work for you and have fun. Laugh it off if it doesn't go right. You're building intimacy and strengthening your relationship by just trying!

Foreplay

We've established that foreplay is of paramount importance. Foreplay goes far beyond a couple of kisses and a bit of fondling. With proper attention and care, foreplay will stoke the furnace of your desire and offer the opportunity to be fully present in the moment. With our busy lives, it isn't easy to just flip a switch and be ready for hot and heavy sex. Foreplay is the transition into sex. So relax and let it develop. Let your desire guide you and revel in the slow, sensual pleasure of foreplay.

Position 1 - Cock's Cradle

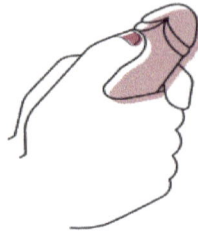

Often the focus is on a single hand stroking the penis in a down motion. With this foreplay position, grab the penis with both hands, cradling it with your thumbs on the underside. For a comfortable grip, you'll need to kneel beside him or even lay between his legs. Massage the penis gently with your thumbs from the root to the tip. Pay particular attention to the base of the head where it joins the shaft. Look at your partner while you massage him to build intimacy and judge your pressure.

Position 2 - Milkmaid

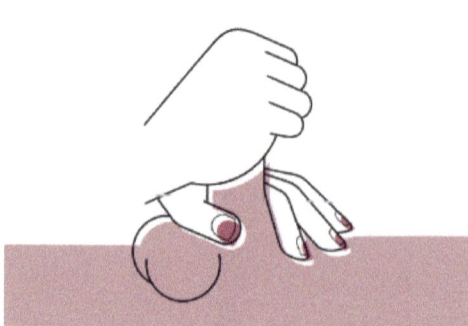

This is another excellent position for pleasuring him while looking at his face and watching his reactions. Hold his eyes as you grasp the base of the penis with one hand, and with the other, stroke up from the bottom and then cover the tip before sliding back down. Use steady, firm pressure with a little squeeze at the top, reminiscent of milking a cow. Don't worry if you've never milked a cow (nobody else has either since the turn of the century!). Just watch your partner's reactions, and adjust your pressure and speed accordingly. A bit of lube is a good idea for this one. You can use massage oil, K-Y, or if you're comfortable with it, get him nice and wet using your mouth. You'll want to be positioned looking toward his head and kneel beside him or between his legs. You can even lie on your stomach if that is comfortable, but your arms won't have as much range of motion like you would if you were kneeling.

Position 3 - Over-Under

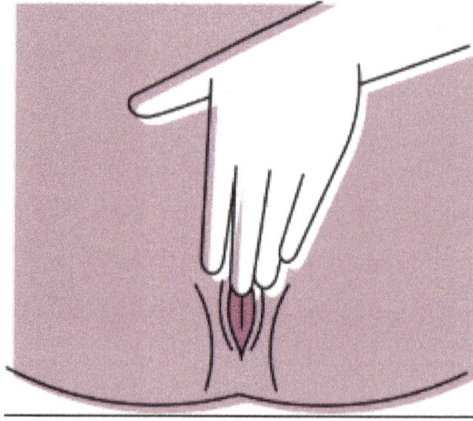

Let's turn the attention to the ladies. This can be done by either you or your partner. Don't underestimate how erotic it is for him to watch you pleasure yourself. While you probably know exactly how to pleasure yourself to achieve orgasm, this is just to get you revved up and ready. Remember, we're talking appetizers, not the main course.

Using one or two fingers, slide slowly up and down the labia, slipping just inside the vagina on the downward stroke. Your goal isn't deep penetration. It is a teasing, light stroke, designed to get the juices flowing and the sensations rolling. As you slide up, vary how far up you go. Sometimes, stimulate the clitoris, and at other times, avoid it. Lubrication should be used to increase pleasure and prevent friction.

This can be done lying side by side while kissing and your bodies touching, or your partner can be completely separate either watching or providing the pleasure while focused on observing your reactions. Either way is highly erotic and intimate. Try not to let shyness take hold. Don't check your reactions. Let him see your pleasure, and share it with you.

Position 4 - Mons Massage

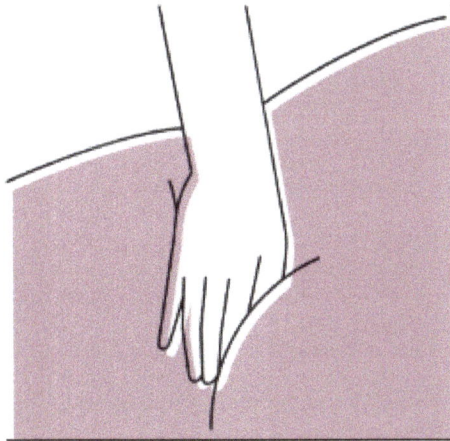

Mons Massage can be done by you or your partner. Indirect pressure to the clitoris is the goal. It also increases blood flow to the area and can heighten the sensations when direct stimulation is applied. The Mons Massage is also a good position if you are super sensitive, and direct stimulation to the clitoris is too intense. You or your partner will massage your mons, also known as your pubic mound, using downward pressure over your clit. Move the pressure around a bit, and massage the labia with sideways pressure on the clitoris. Try different motions- circles, up/down, side-to-side. Mons Massage is a bit like taking the scenic route to get somewhere. Relax and enjoy the journey!

Here are a few last notes on foreplay before we move on. Don't rush through it. Linger over it like you're savoring a good meal or watching a beautiful sunset. Let it find its own way, and avoid falling into patterns. Try new things regularly to keep it spontaneous and exciting. Don't only focus on the standard erogenous zones. Explore each other. You might find a delicious spot on your partner's left shoulder or behind their right knee that you never knew was there that makes them quiver with pleasure. Finally, you don't have to be in the bedroom to start foreplay. Meaningful glances, flirting, a stolen kiss in the kitchen, or holding hands on the couch are all great starts. Let it build into an inferno before taking it to the bedroom: tease each other with caresses, indulge in a quick make-out session in the pantry, whisper in his ear something that you're looking forward to, or even send a flirty email or text message to set the mood before you're even in the same room. The sky's the limit when it comes to foreplay. Let your imagination run wild, and enjoy the ride!

Oral Sex

Before we go any further, we need to dispel some myths and banish some demons. Oral sex can be incredibly pleasurable but incredibly daunting to many people. First of all, there is nothing gross about it. If you are focused on bodily fluids, your mind isn't on the pleasure that you are getting or giving. Focus on the sensations, not on biology.

Another common barrier to enjoying oral sex is the ultra-intimate contact. Concerns about physical appearance, smell, and taste can plague the recipient, blocking their ability to enjoy themselves. If your partner wants to do it, then they aren't worried about these things. They want to give you pleasure and enjoy your reactions. They find it erotic, and most certainly are not there to judge if something is too big, too small, or whatever your particular concern is. They are there to drive you wild and get turned on right along with you.

A few tips for enjoying and giving oral pleasure:

Be clean- This is one of the biggest worries. A fresh shower or a quick wash-up can help you relax and enjoy.

Enjoy the spotlight- While oral pleasure can be enjoyed simultaneously, most often one person is giving, and the other is receiving. This undivided attention can be uncomfortable for the receiver because all the focus is on them. It also can set up a tit for tat scenario where one partner feels pressure to reciprocate for the pleasure they received. Try to shut your brain off, and get lost in sensations. Sex and pleasure are not a contest, and you are not being judged. Enjoy your moment, and let the next steps unfold how they will.

Open your eyes- Watching your partner during oral sex is profoundly intimate. When possible, meet their eyes, and let them see your pleasure and excitement. Whether giving or receiving, eye contact adds a layer of eroticism that you'll sadly miss if your shutters are drawn tight!

Position 5 - The Basic Blow

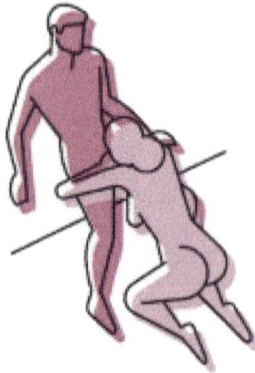

Alright, let's talk technique for a moment. Whether he's standing, lying, or sitting, the basic idea is the same. Take his penis in your mouth, and slide it in and out. You control how far into your mouth or throat you take it. If you've got a sensitive gag reflex, keep it shallow. If you can take it deep, slide the tip of the penis to the back of your throat and go through the motions of swallowing. The action of the throat muscles around the head of his penis will definitely get you a groan or two.

You don't have to go extremely fast with the in and out motion. Take your time especially in the beginning. You'll want to suck a bit as well, particularly when you are pulling your mouth up or away from your partner's body. Adding some suction toward the end of that motion as you reach the tip will make his toes curl.

Don't forget to use your tongue, too. Release him from your mouth, and lick his penis like you would an ice cream cone. Don't forget the testicles. Some men really like having their scrotums licked, sucked, or fondled while you work his shaft with your hand or mouth. For others, it can be too sensitive. Go easy to begin with, and see what his reaction is before being too aggressive with "the boys."

Finally, you can add your hand if you really want to drive him wild. Firmly stroke him with your hand in tandem with your mouth. The pressure of your hand along with the warm moistness of your mouth is a match made in heaven. You can add a bit of a twist with your hand as you stroke and vary the amount of pressure. You'll have him on the edge in no time.

Position 6 - The Stinger

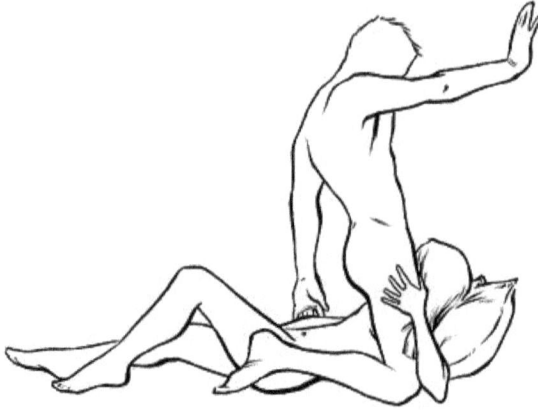

You'll love getting stung in this position. Lie back, but prop yourself up with some pillows. You'll want some decent support under your neck and shoulders. This position works well on the couch too. Your partner will straddle your chest just under your arms. You'll want your arms free so you can use your hand as discussed in Position 5. Take his penis in your mouth, and move your head back and forth, running your mouth up and down his shaft. This can be a bit of a neck workout, but he can help by thrusting his hips. Don't be afraid to tell him if he is thrusting too deep or hard. Just take it easy on your neck to avoid straining it. The stinger can be incredibly intimate and erotic. Look up and watch his face as you pleasure him. This position affords him a great view of you and his penis in your mouth- a definite turn-on for any guy.

Position 7 - The Honey Pot

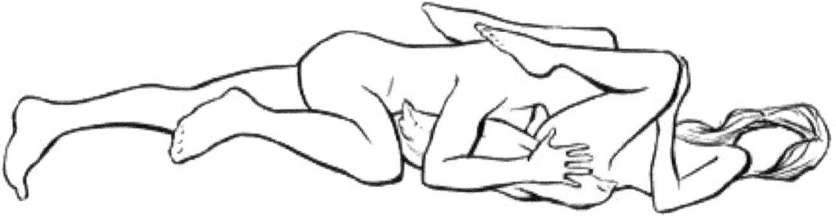

For this position, lay back and relax. Easier said than done sometimes, but this is your time. Try to get out of your head. Your partner is not worried about if your thighs are too big. Their focus is your pleasure; make sure it's your focus too. You can put some pillows under your hips to give them a bit of a better angle as well. Your partner can lie between your legs on his stomach or kneel beside you. Kneeling next to you can have the added bonus of giving you access to his penis to stroke or even just a light caress on his butt and legs.

Your partner will use his tongue to stimulate the clitoris. Sucking back against the area can be intensely pleasurable as well. Spread the labia apart, or push up on the mons to help pull back the clitoral hood to increase direct contact with the clitoris. If you are extremely sensitive, this might be too much so go easy at first. Bend your knees, and draw them toward your shoulders to also offer better access as well. Experiment with your leg positions until you find something that is comfortable and rocks your world.

Don't be afraid to let him know what you like. Rock your hips or circle them in a rhythm against his mouth for added sensation. An extra tip for him. In addition to his mouth, encourage him to use his fingers as well. Slipping a finger or two inside your vagina as he works your clitoris with his mouth is guaranteed to escalate your pleasure. He can make the 'come here' motion with his fingers inside the vagina to stimulate your G-spot and send you into orbit.

Position 8 - Dining at the 'Y'

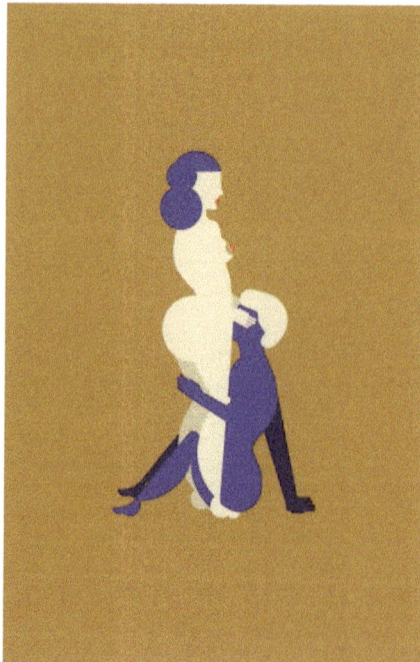

Standing to receive oral pleasure might feel a bit strange at first. However, it offers an excellent change in angles and view for you. Consider leaning against the wall for support. The clitoral stimulation will not be as intense as if you are lying down with your legs wide. Widen your stance as you stand in this position to give your partner the best access. You can also round your lower back slightly to tip your hips up. This is the perfect position to caress his head or bury your fingers in his hair. This position is a great one for the shower or a quickie in a tight space.

Position 9 - The Hovering Flower

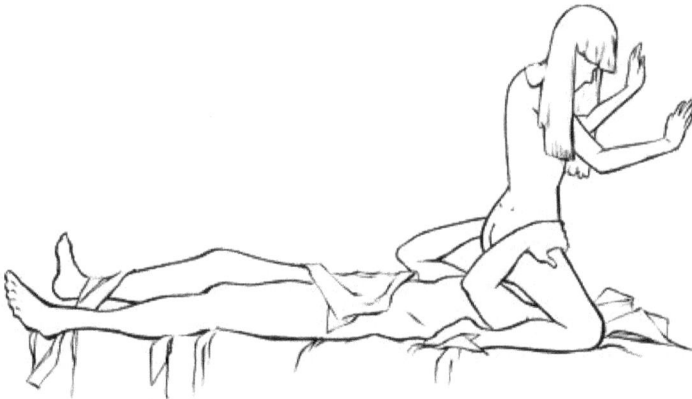

This position can be intimidating to many women. Your partner lies back, and you position yourself over his face by straddling his head. Simple enough, but many times women get caught up in their minds during this one. They worry about if their thighs are jiggling, or if their partner can breathe. These are definitely counter-intuitive to enjoying all of the amazing rewards this position offers. First, have confidence that men find this position highly erotic. Your thighs are the furthest things from their mind. From there, lower yourself to his mouth. Brace yourself against a wall or the bed frame for support, and let sensation guide you from there. Rock or circle your hips, or raise and lower yourself for different pressures.

Position 10 - 69

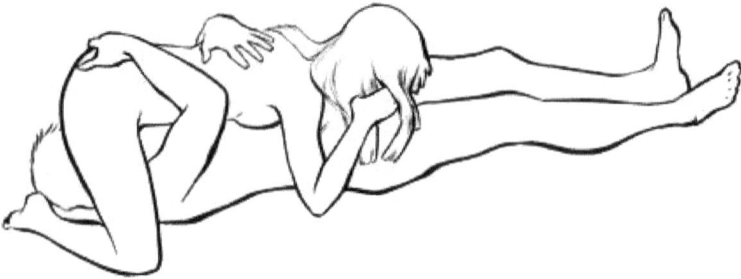

We didn't miscount! The famed 69 position is one of the most famous of all sex positions. Named because the partners are joined together like the 6 and the 9 in the number 69, this position is highly erotic and intimate. It can be done with either partner on top but is most commonly performed with the woman on top. To achieve this position (ladies on top), your partner lies flat on his back, and you straddle his face, looking toward his feet. Lean forward so you can take his penis in your mouth. This position can be difficult if there is a considerable height difference in partners. You can vary this position by laying on your sides which can work well if there are knee issues for either partner. The man on top variation can be fun as well; just make sure you have enough room to control the depth of his penis in your mouth. It can get tiresome on your neck if you're doing a lot of up and down motions. If your neck is getting tired, take a rest, and use your hand or tongue for awhile.

Vaginal Sex

The next fifty or so positions are dedicated to vaginal sex. It is the most common form of sexual acts and tends to fall into predictable patterns. While every time you and your partner have sex doesn't need to be an all-out athletic event with multiple position changes, the more you experiment and try new things, the more you'll enjoy it. It keeps things fresh and exciting. It'll keep your sex life from slowly slipping down your priority list because it has become ho-hum and not worth the effort.

Position 11 - The Classic Missionary

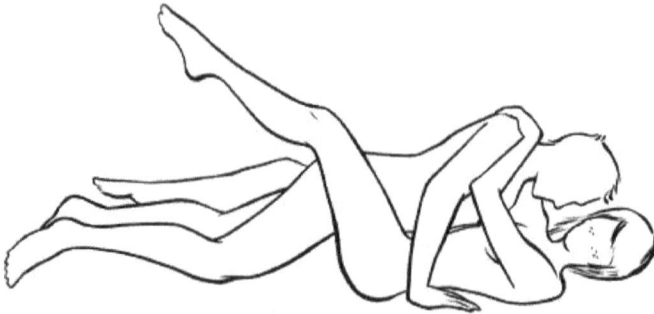

It only makes sense to start with the most basic of all sexual positions. This classic is tried and true and often gets a bad rap of being "boring." To get into the position, you lie on your back, and your partner positions himself over you between your legs, entering you from the front. He thrusts his hips, creating an in and out motion inside your vagina. Missionary Position is an excellent position to build intimacy as you are face-to-face; it doesn't have to be overly vigorous, and allows for lots of extra touching, kissing, and skin-to-skin contact. It also provides the opportunity for him to play with your breasts while giving you a good view of him doing it.

Missionary doesn't have to be boring, though. Ladies, do not be tempted just to lie there, and let your partner do all the work. Rock your hips, meeting his thrusts, or even make circles with your pelvis. You can also take your legs and wrap them around his lower leg so your ankles and calves are resting on his. The movement of your legs changes the angle of your hips and will produce a different sensation. Take the opportunity to explore his back and butt with your hands. Another tip to add spice to your missionary position is play with the tempo. How slow can you go? Concentrate on the sensations as you move in slow motion. Pick up the speed for a grand finish. One final tip, pile pillows up to elevate your hips to change the angle of entry for different sensations.

Position 12 - Here Kitty

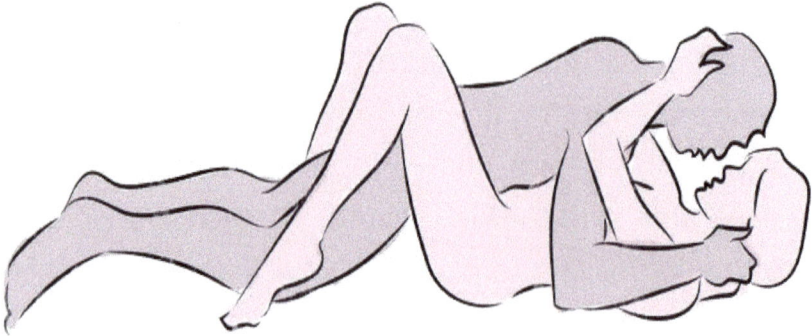

This position is a variation of the missionary featuring a technique called clitoral alignment technique or CAT. The goal of this position is to increase clitoral stimulation which is something that the missionary position doesn't offer. Again, you are on your back, and your partner is on top between your legs. This time, you need to bend your knees, and plant your feet on the bed. Your partner positions himself further up on your torso than in missionary position. Your partner's chest should be closer to your shoulders, and he will be slightly off to one side. The thrusting motion is more up and down than in and out, but experiment with hip motions to get the most stimulation as possible. Vaginal orgasms can be challenging for a lot of women, but this will significantly increase the odds of reaching orgasm by adding in the clitoral stimulation.

Position 13 - Twister

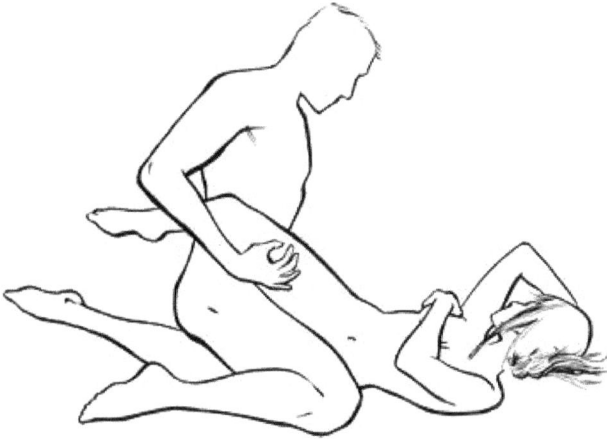

This position allows for very deep penetration, but keeps you and your partner face to face. You'll lie on your side. Your partner straddles your leg on the bed, and you wrap your upper leg around him. He can help support your upper leg by pinning it to his body. Keep your shoulders flat on the bed, putting you in a perfect position for him to play with your breasts as well as stimulate your clit while he thrusts. Twister offers you a great view of your partner. Don't waste it. Keep your eyes open and watch! Feel free to pinch your nipples or rock your hips in time with him. You will need to have enough flexibility in your hips and back to twist yourself and allow him to move.

Position 14 - Scissors

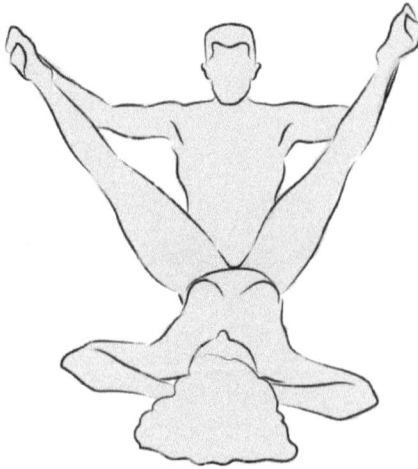

This position requires a bit of flexibility, particularly in your hips and inner thighs. In this position, you are again on your back. This time, put your legs straight in the air, and let them fall open. Your partner kneels close to your butt and grasps your ankles. As he enters you and beings to thrust his hips, open and close your legs. He should help by supporting your ankles as you move your legs. It might take a moment, but you'll find a rhythm. Experiment with legs opened vs. legs closed with each thrust to see what feels best. Maintain good communication with your partner so your legs don't get stretched too far for comfort. This position is also fun to do with your partner standing on the floor at the edge of the bed especially if alignment when he is kneeling is problematic. You'll want to get your hips just hanging off of the bed, but not so far that you're about to fall off. You need to be securely supported so you don't hurt your back as you move your legs.

Position 15 - Push-up

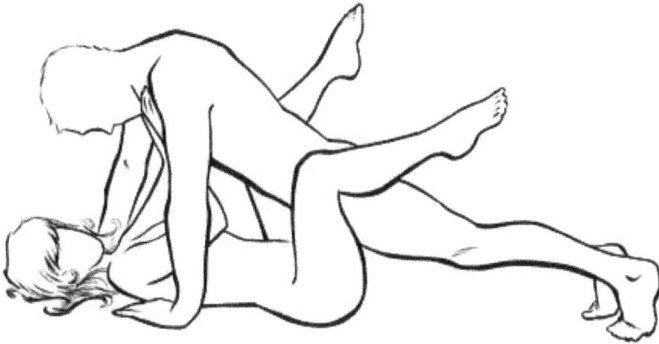

This position is a commanding position for your partner and can be incredibly erotic for you especially if you can relax and hand him the reins for a bit. You lie on your back, and he positions himself between your legs. The critical variation here from the Missionary Position is that he is bearing all of his weight. The primary point of contact is where he is joined with you. From this position, he has full control of the depth and rate. He can tease you with just the tip of his penis, sheath himself deep within you with one powerful thrust, or can pull completely out and enter you over and over again. A mix of these options is guaranteed to drive you wild. You also have room to reach down and stimulate your clit, or roam your hands over his chest and shoulders. The Push-up Position does take a lot of core and upper body strength on his part.

Position 16 - Over the Shoulders

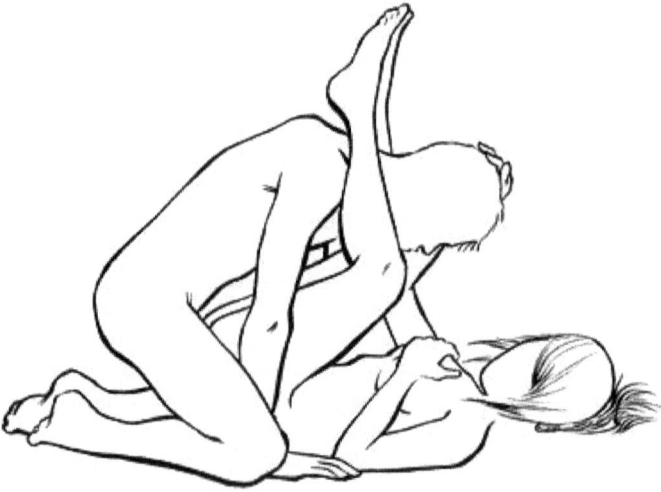

Over the Shoulders position is another position that allows for deep penetration. It also requires quite a bit of flexibility for you in your back and hips. The position requires you to lie on your back and draw your legs up, placing them on your partner's shoulders. As he leans forward, your back rounds, and your pelvis tilts up. The angle of this position allows for G-spot stimulation and can be very intense for both partners. Because of the stress on your legs and hips, ask your partner to start gently and let you get accustomed to the position. If putting your legs on his shoulders is too much for your hips, try your feet to his chest instead. A good way to add an extra layer of pleasure is for him to circle his hips or rock side to side. Once you settle into this position, you can experiment with putting your arms over your head or holding onto the headboard of the bed.

Position 17 - Do the Twist

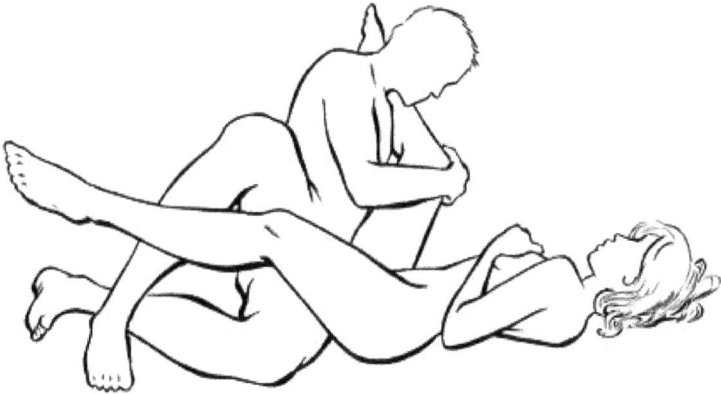

Do the Twist takes a bit of flexibility and strength for your partner. To achieve this position, you'll lie on your back with your legs open and bent at the knee. Your partner positions himself near your butt and places your leg on his shoulder. The thrusting motion is a bit of a twist and might be difficult for a man with back issues. It provides a clear avenue for eye contact and an open position for him to watch your reactions. A great way to add spice is for you to play with your breasts and nipples, or pleasure yourself by rubbing your clitoris. Watching you self-pleasure can be a huge turn-on for your partner. Consider a pillow under your hips if the alignment is difficult.

Position 18 - Lover's Dance

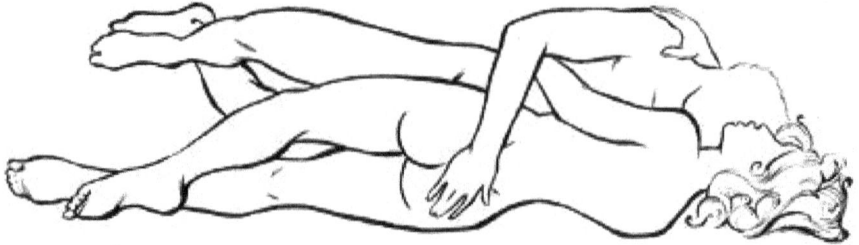

This position is incredibly intimate. It offers full body contact with lots of options for kissing and touching. It doesn't allow for very deep penetration, but with proper alignment, it can provide lots of clitoral stimulation. You simply need to part your legs and allow him to enter you. It isn't meant to be vigorous. Rather, this position is typically done in a slow and gentle manner with the focus on the sensations and intimacy. If penetration is challenging, try draping your upper leg over your partner's hip to get a bit closer. This can be a good position if either partner has a lower extremity injury or other physical limitations. Take your time, and let this position gently build until your passions boil over.

Position 19 - Bear Hug

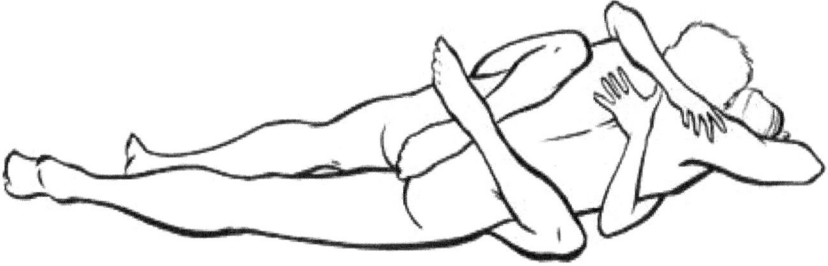

With this position, intimacy is at its maximum. You lie on your side and open your arms and legs. Your partner will lie facing you on top of your lower leg and arm. You will then wrap both of your arms and legs around your partner. You should try to hook your ankles together, if possible. Depending on the size of you and your partner, this might be too much weight on your lower leg and arm. You can roll onto your back slightly, pulling him more onto your body, and he can bear some of his weight on his arm to help alleviate any discomfort for you. This position allows for deeper penetration while getting as close as possible with as much contact as possible. Rock together, and enjoy the sensation of being as closely joined together as you can possibly be.

Position 20 - The X-Games

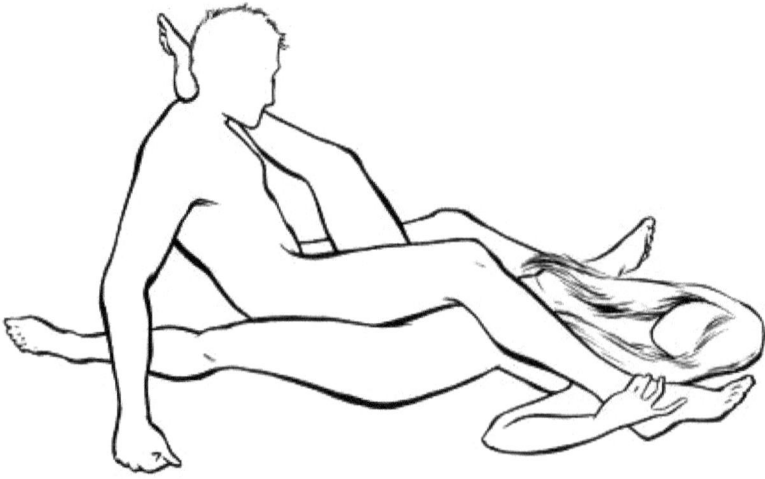

This one isn't nearly as hard as it looks. Face each other on the bed. Ladies, open your legs, lean back, and let your partner slide up between them. Lay one leg over his leg, and take his leg across your torso to the shoulder. The depth of penetration will depend significantly on individual flexibility, but it will likely be relatively shallow. The X-Games concentrates a lot of stimulation on the tip of the penis and the vaginal opening, both extraordinarily erotic and sensitive areas. Thrusting is replaced by more of a rocking or a gyrating motion. You should have a free hand and adequate access for clitoral stimulation for added excitement and to help achieve orgasm.

Position 21 - Spider Swing

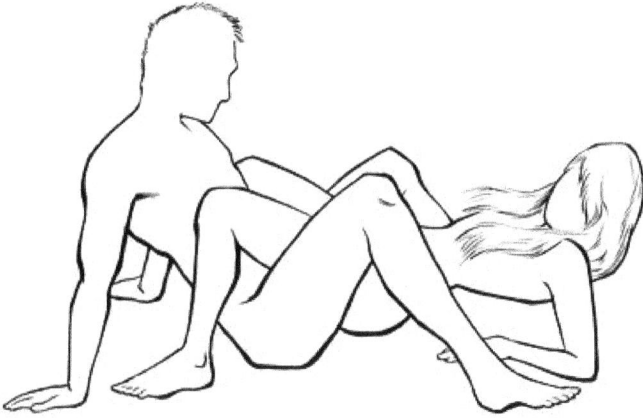

This position is a great way to explore new angles. While you face each other, your partner opens his legs. You slide between his legs and slip your legs over the top of his, planting them on either side of his hips. Move closer, and guide him inside you. This posture can give either partner a great view of him entering you. You can lift and lower your hips, or you can rock together. Sometimes, pillows under your hips or shoulders can give added support. Again, this is not a position with hard thrusting. It does offer an excellent opportunity for eye contact, breast play, or clitoral stimulation. This one can require a decent amount of strength and flexibility to hold for a long time.

Position 22 - Belly Flop

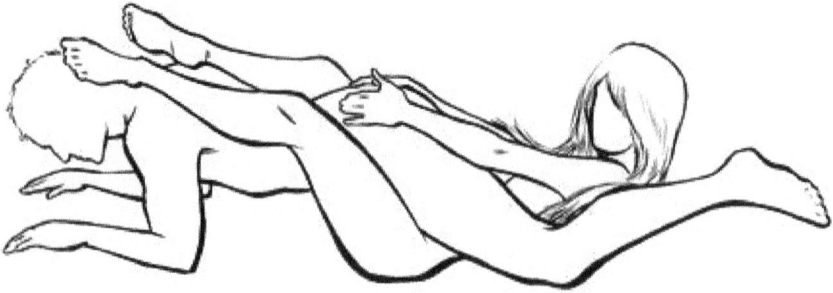

While not a terribly intimate position, this position offers one of the most unique angles and views of all the positions. You'll lie on your back and open your legs. Your partner will face away from you as he lies on top of you. Prop your legs on his shoulders while he supports his weight on his forearms. Propping your legs up tilts your pelvis up and helps meet his downward thrusts. This allows for a lot of clitoral stimulation and gives you a chance to admire his backside. If you want to watch the show, you can prop yourself up on pillows to elevate your shoulders and support your neck. Take the opportunity to massage and caress his butt and thighs. You can also lightly stimulate his perineum (the skin between the base of his scrotum and his anus). Go easy at first, and get feedback before you get too aggressive in this region. Some guys love it, and others find it too intense.

Position 23 - The Classic Cowgirl

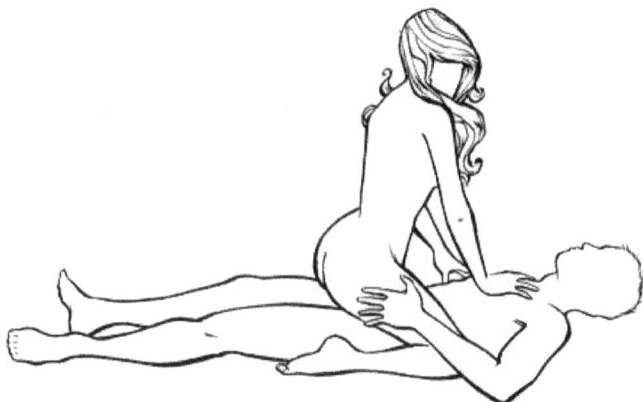

The Classic Cowgirl is in the top three most used sexual positions. It is the go-to woman on top position and for good reason. Deep penetration and highly erotic views for him and you are both benefits of this position. To achieve this position, your partner lies on his back, and you straddle his hips. You'll then rock your hips or bounce up and down on his penis. Depending on how tall you are and how big he is, you can either be on your knees or keep your feet flat on the bed and squat down onto him. The squatting method is quite a workout, and you'll need a lot of leg strength to keep it up for long.

Many women love the freedom and control offered in this position. It can be difficult for some women with hip or knee issues and takes a bit of stamina to maintain for long. It does allow for clitoral stimulation by either you or your partner. It can be highly intimate with good eye contact, but other things like kissing and a lot of skin-to-skin contact are lacking. It is one of the highest rated positions among men so give it a try and stay in the saddle for as long as you can!

Position 24 - The Butterfly

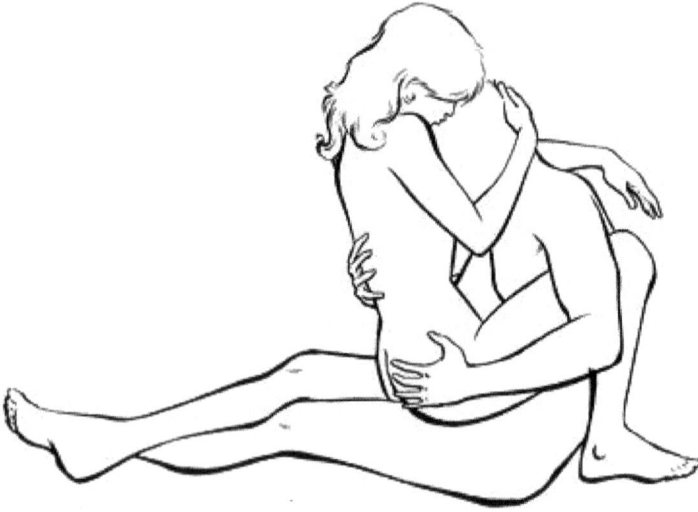

This position gets top marks for intimacy. It is incredibly close, and allows for a lot of eye contact, kissing, and skin against skin. Have your partner sit with his legs outstretched. It is best to be propped up by pillows against the wall or bed frame to support his back. Straddle his hips and lower yourself onto him by squatting down. Allow your weight to rest in his lap. This position is good for slow, sensual exploration and connection. A gentle rocking motion is more appropriate than trying to bounce vigorously. You or he can stimulate your clit while you move. This one can be tough for people with back issues. It requires core strength on your part since you don't have any back support.

Position 25 - Cowboy Up

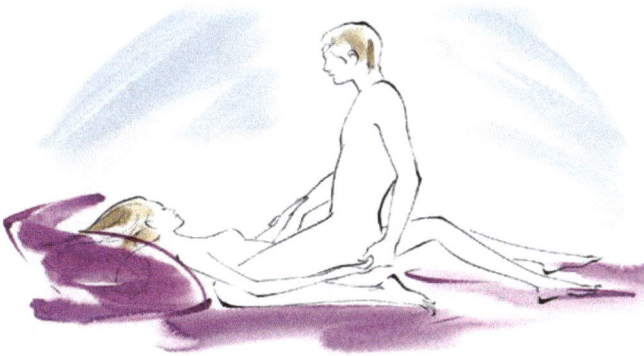

Ready for a very different rodeo? In this position, your partner straddles your hips while you lay flat. Since your legs are mostly closed, penetration will not be overly deep, but it will be quite intense for him due to the tighter fit. This position is highly intimate. It allows you to touch and explore him, and your breasts are clear for him to play with. Good eye contact is another bonus.

Position 26 - The Link

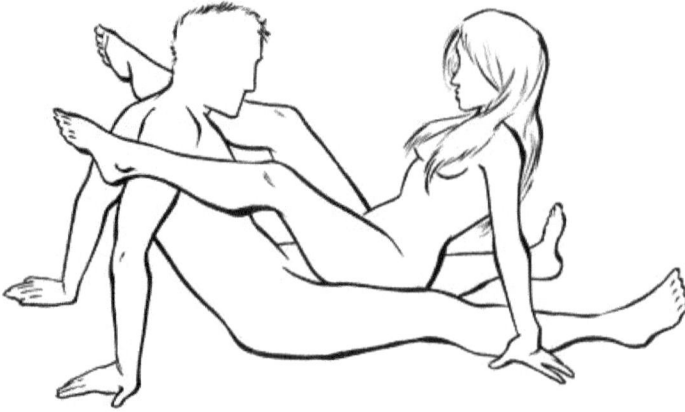

This position can be slightly challenging because it does require you to have a good deal of flexibility. Your partner will sit with his legs open wide and lean back on his arms. He'll need to be reclining slightly, but can be propped up with some pillows against the wall or bed frame. You'll slide yourself onto him, and lean back so you can put your legs on his shoulders. The depth of penetration depends a lot on your flexibility. If you're having trouble with alignment, add a pillow under your butt to lift you up. You're in control of the movement. Grind your hips or rock back and forth for different sensations. You're also in a great position to receive clitoral stimulation. You can also have good eye contact, and he is treated to a beautiful view of your breasts and face with this position.

Position 27 - Waterfall

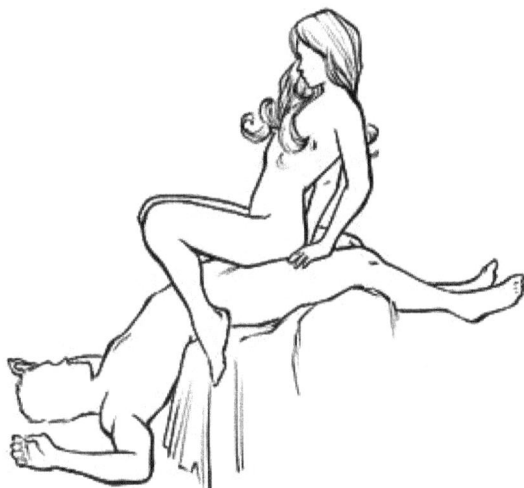

This advanced position requires balance, flexibility, and strength on your part. Your partner arranges himself on the edge of the bed, and his torso drapes down to the floor. His shoulders should touch the floor. If he has any neck or lower back problems, this position won't work well. You straddle his hips and lower yourself onto him. Brace yourself with your hands behind you on his thighs and your feet on the edge of the bed. You are in complete control of the movement and can rock or bounce. Intimacy is not the focus of this position. It offers deep penetration, unusual angles and motions, and a tantalizing view particularly for him. Don't be afraid to rest and give him a show while you pleasure yourself by rubbing your clit or playing with your breasts.

Position 28 - Lap Dance

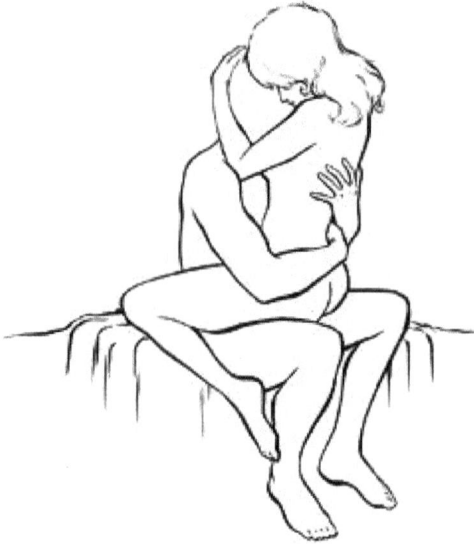

This highly erotic and intimate posture allows for exploration of the places on your shoulders and neck that drive you wild. An excellent position for good skin-to-skin contact, holding each other's gaze, and kissing, the Lap Dance is designed to be done on the edge of the bed or in a chair. Your partner should have his feet on the floor. You will straddle his hips by kneeling on the bed. If he is in a chair, keep your feet on the floor and use a squatting motion, if you're tall enough. It offers deep penetration, and you will be in control of the tempo. This does require a decent amount of leg strength to sustain though your partner can help support your back. He can also aid the motion by rocking his hips, or using his hands on your butt or hips to give you an extra boost. Don't be afraid to take a break from moving, and just enjoy touching and kissing your partner while he is seated deep within you.

Position 29 - Bottoms Up

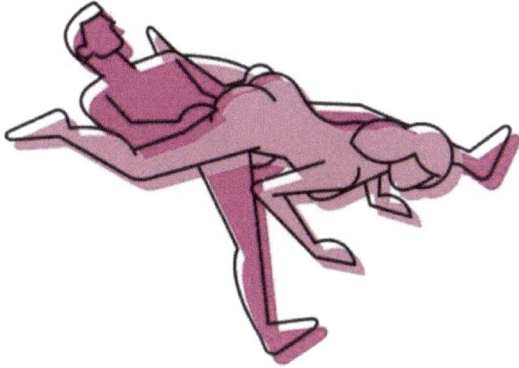

This position requires a good deal of flexibility and strength. It offers a unique angle and a different view for your partner. Your partner lays flat with his legs open, and you straddle his hips before lowering your upper body between his legs. You should be down closer to his feet, and your motion will be more of a rocking from back and forth rather than up and down. Achieving proper alignment and entry can be a challenge with this position. Try starting from the reverse cowgirl position (#47 for reference) if you are having troubles. This is not a very intimate position, and penetration is usually shallow, focusing the stimulation on the tip of the penis and the entrance to your vagina.

Position 30 - Row Your Boat

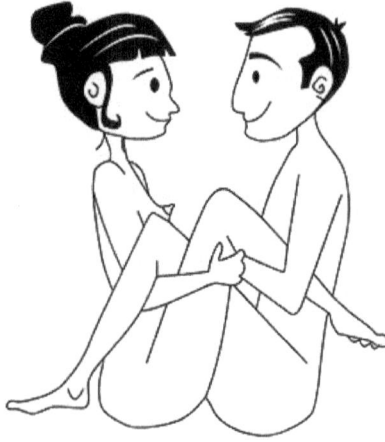

This position will have you singing *Row, Row, Row Your Boat Gently up My Stream* in no time. Using the boat pose from yoga, you and your partner will come together in a whole new way. To achieve this position, first you'll straddle your partner's hips and lower yourself onto him just like in Classic Cowgirl. He then sits up, and you'll slide back off of his hips and onto your butt. Both of you bend your knees and thread your arms under the other's knees. Both of your feet, as well as your partner's, should be off the ground and your weight balanced on your butt. Find a comfy handhold, and begin to rock back and forth. Row Your Boat can be a little tricky at first, but once you get your rhythm established, you can experiment with different leg positions. Try putting your legs on his shoulders or putting your feet on the ground. This does take a good bit of flexibility and strength to achieve but not an extreme amount. Take breaks to kiss and touch each other to extend your time in this position.

Position 31 - The Seesaw

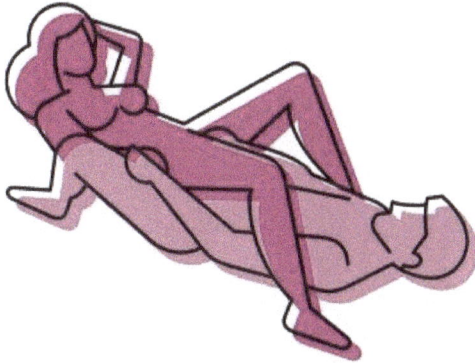

This position offers a lot of variations and requires you and your partner to work together. To start, you will straddle your partner and squat down, lowering yourself onto him. Let your weight rest against him and reposition your feet to either side of his shoulders. From here, you can stay sitting upright, and rock back and forth. You'll be wide open for either one of you to rub your clitoris, and the gentle rocking with deep penetration can be highly pleasurable. You can change it up by leaning back between his legs. You can either prop yourself up with your hands behind your back, or you can grab your partner's hands and move with a kind of push/pull motion. This requires quite a bit of core strength for both of you. If you've got the flexibility, you can lay all the way back between his legs, and he can grab your hips to control the motions. Finally, your partner can draw his knees up behind your back, and you can lean back against them. This will lead to a more shallow penetration, but can be highly intimate as he cradles you with his body while inside you.

Position 32 - The "L"

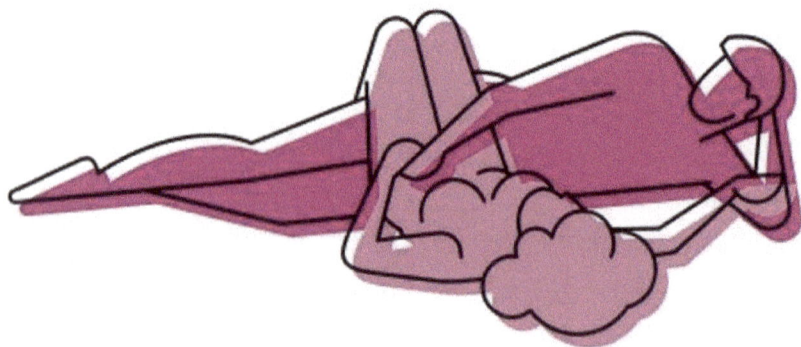

The "L" is all about the angle. You and your partner will make a 90-degree angle just like the capital "L". Your partner will lie on his side, and you'll arrange yourself perpendicular to him. Drape your legs over his hips. The penetration on this one is not deep, and the movement is mostly from him making a twisting, rocking motion with his hips. This is a gentle position, and because you can have good eye contact and your hands can roam freely is highly intimate as well. For a variation, you lay on your side with your knees drawn up to a 90-degree angle like you're sitting in a chair. Your partner kneels close to your butt and thighs, making an upright "L" with your bodies. Depending on height, alignment can be tricky so use pillows under your hips or one between your legs to help. Penetration will be deeper with this variation, but the intimacy and gentleness of the posture are lost.

Position 33 - Riding Sidesaddle

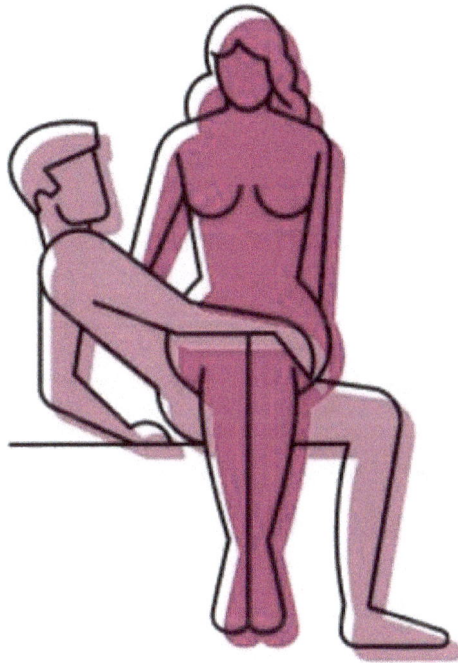

The sidesaddle is really best done in a chair, either a recliner or a chair with no arms. Your partner sits with his feet on the floor, and you sit on his lap sideways. You'll control the movements by pushing up with your arms and legs and lifting your hips. It requires both upper and lower body strength as well as core strength. Your partner can thrust a bit with his hips by pushing off of the floor and lifting his pelvis. Penetration will vary, but there are lots of opportunities for kissing, fondling, or clitoral stimulation.

Position 34 - Rocking Horse

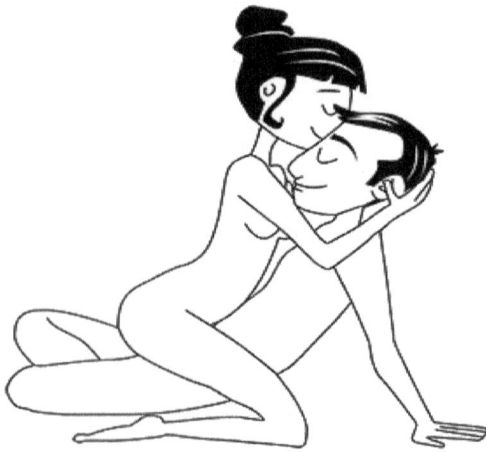

This position allows for more body contact than the Classic Cowgirl and can be a bit easier on your knees and hips. On the flip side, it requires more flexibility for your partner through his knees and hips. Your partner will sit cross-legged and lean back a bit. This brings his pelvis up and will make penetration easier for you without requiring quite as much bend in your knees and hips. You'll straddle his hips and lower yourself on to him. You can lean back or move straight up and down. For extra stimulation, slide your torso along his as you raise yourself upright on your knees. Be careful as you come back down that he is aligned properly especially if you are moving quickly. The Rocking Horse is a highly intimate position with lots of eye contact and opportunities for kissing and caressing.

Position 35 - The Swing

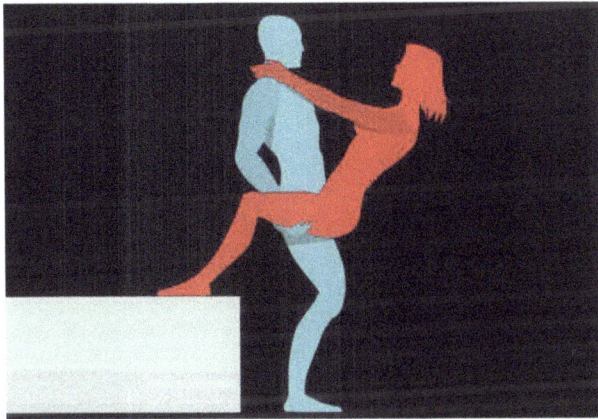

This position feels a bit like movie star sex. It requires a lot of core strength from both parties, and there are obvious limitations if you are much bigger than your partner. However, there are ways to make this one a bit more manageable. To achieve the position, your partner lifts you onto him while you wrap your arms and legs around him. To help support some of your weight, see if you can find something to brace your feet on. Then you can wrap your arms around his neck or grab his shoulders for leverage. This can be hard on your partner's back so this is not a good idea for anyone with back issues. Your grip can get uncomfortable on his neck and shoulders as well so be mindful of that.

Position 36 - Cum to the Kitchen

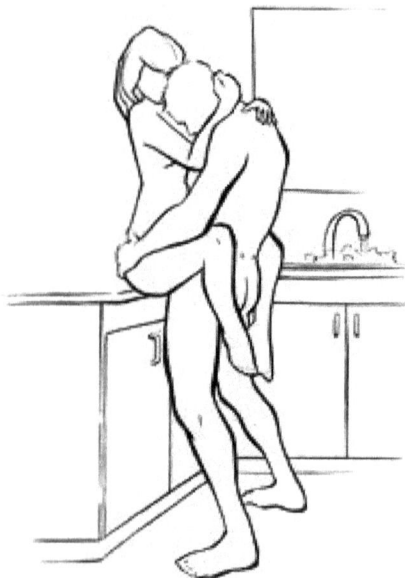

What could be more erotic than sex on the kitchen counter? The element of excitement from the seduction and passion that just won't be contained until you get to the bedroom adds heat to this position. Since your weight is born by the counter, the need for Incredible Hulk strength is not needed. Height can be an issue, depending on how high your counter is versus how tall your partner is. A small step for him or a pillow under your butt can help adjust the heights. Hop up on the counter, and slide yourself to the very edge. Your partner will stand between your legs, and you can wrap your arms and legs around him.

Position 37 - Stand to Attention

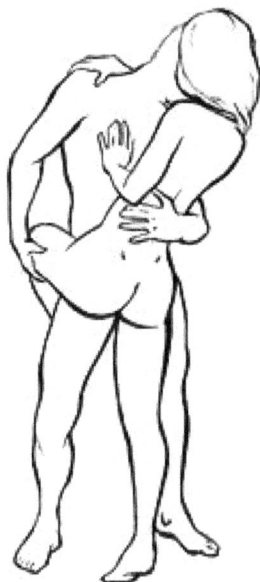

This standing position is ideal for close quarters, showers, closets, or anywhere where else that the mood strikes, and there is no handy bed in sight. Height differences are the main issue with this position but can be overcome with a little ingenuity. To achieve this position, you'll raise one leg and wrap it around your partner's hip, allowing him to slide into you from the front. It typically isn't very deep penetration, and you'll need a good amount of strength in your standing leg and core to pull it off. He can help support your raised leg by pinning it to his hip. This is an intimate position and is perfect for eye contact and kissing.

Position 38 - The Bridge

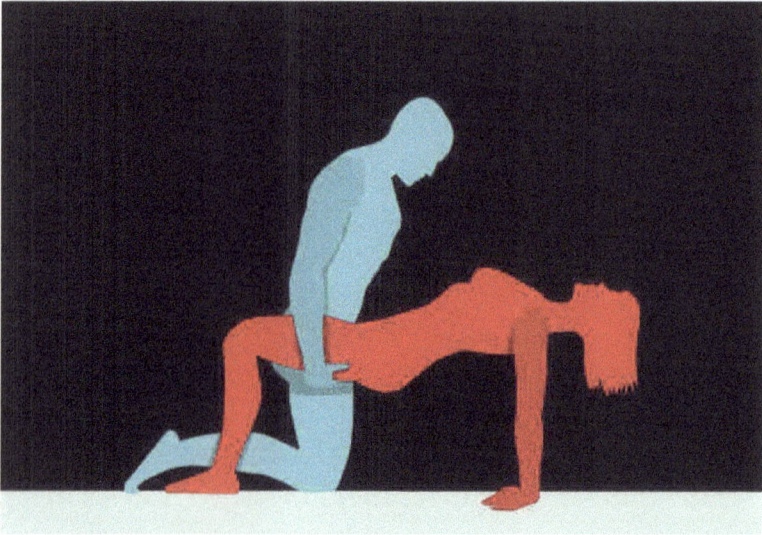

The bridge position requires a good deal of strength on your part. However, a great way to achieve this position but get some extra support is to use an exercise ball or even a small ottoman would work under your upper back. You just need to be able to support your upper body and allow your hips to swing freely. Your partner will kneel between your legs, and grab each thigh to help support your hips. You can control the motion by rocking back and forth on your arms, or he can thrust and pull you onto him. The key to this position is to let yourself move as easily as possible. Deep penetration and powerful thrusts are definite benefits to this position. It can be tough on your neck as well.

Position 39 – Head Rush

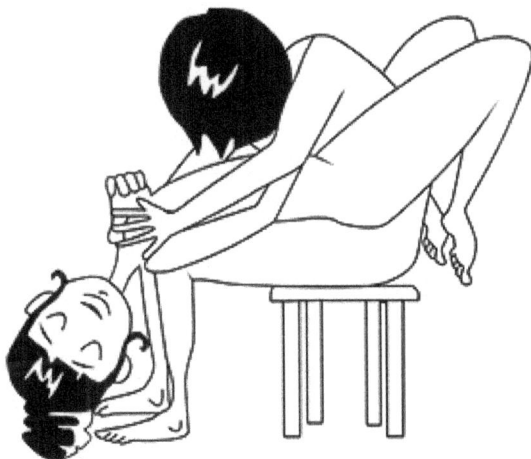

This position will leave you dizzy with the rush of blood to your head on top of the pleasure between your legs. Head Rush can be done sitting on a chair or the edge of the bed. It might not be a bad idea to put a cushion on the floor under your head, just in case. Your partner will sit on the chair or the edge of the bed. You'll straddle his hips and wrap your legs around his waist. Let yourself fall backward (in a controlled fall!). Depending on your situation, you might need to be balanced by grabbing his hands or some other handhold. If you're secure in your position, just open your body to him and let him control the motions. You'll need to be flexible in your back and hips to be comfortable in this position. This is a highly erotic posture for him. You are wrapped around him and open to him at the same time. Encourage him to touch and explore as you enjoy the head rush and lose yourself in pleasure.

Position 40 - T-Bone

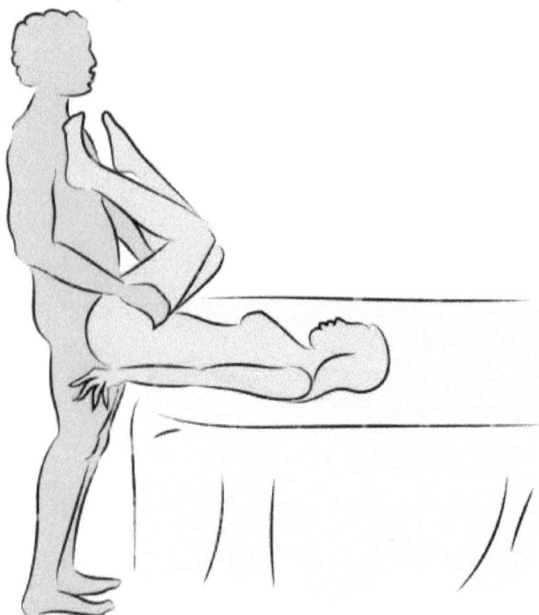

This position is a good position for deep penetration and is usually a favorite for the men. He will stand at the edge of the bed. You slide to where you're just about to fall off the edge, and then lift your legs to his chest or shoulders. You'll need a bit of flexibility, but your knees can be bent if you have tight hamstrings. If you're able to draw your legs back toward your shoulders and tilt your pelvis even further, you can change the angle of entry for different sensations. This position gives him a great view of him sliding into you, of your breasts, and of your face. You can play with your nipples or clit for added stimulation.

Position 41 - Water Sports

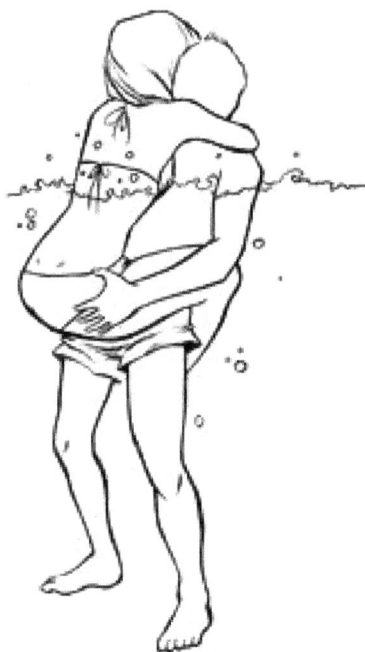

Sex in the water can be a lot of fun. The buoyancy from the water can help achieve different positions from what might be possible on dry land. Before going any further, you must ensure your safety first. Water can be dangerous so be sensible and know your limitations. Sex in the water can also be done discreetly with minor wardrobe adjustments so there is an opportunity for that very private and intimate connection in a public place. Just use good judgment! Also, sex in the water should be done in clean water. You'll end up with quite a bit of water inside your vagina so if it isn't clean, you could wind up with an infection.

Simply wrap your legs around your partner's hips and draw him into you. You can rock or bounce, or he can lift you aided by the buoyancy of the water. Different levels of water can lead to different variations. For example, in water that reaches your partner's hips, you can float on your back, and he can thrust into you and push and pull you on and off of him at the same time. Water offers a degree of freedom for couples that struggle with varying their positions in the bedroom.

Position 42 - Banana Split

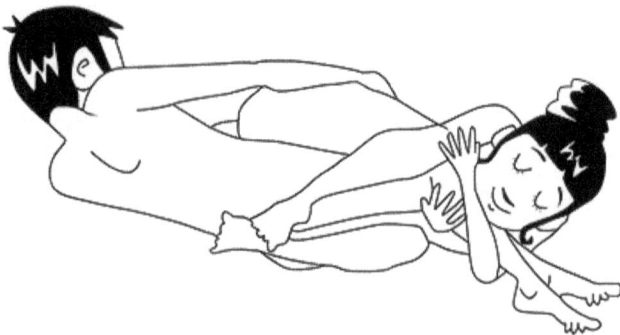

This one looks a bit strange at first, but it a very unique way to experience a different angle of penetration. It also offers the bonus that neither partner needs to be bearing their weight on their upper body or on their knees. To achieve this position, your partner will lie on his side, and you'll lie facing him but with your head to his feet. He'll slide between your legs, so his legs will drape over your bottom leg. Wrap your arms and legs around his legs, and together, you'll rock back and forth. From this angle, his shaft will slide along your clit as he moves in and out of you. The drawback of this position is that your face is close to his feet which can be very unsexy for some people. A blanket or a towel can hide them from view if you find them distracting or unappealing.

Position 43 - Hoist My Sail

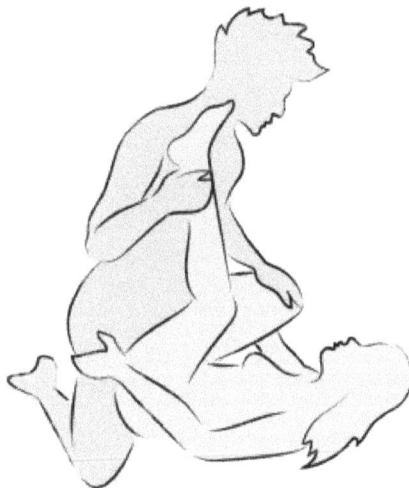

In this position, your legs will make an "L" or look like the mast of a ship. Lie on your back and put one leg straight up. Draw your partner into you by wrapping your other leg around his hip. If you have the flexibility, he can lean forward and thrust himself in a downward angle. This can lead to very deep penetration, and you are also open for fondling and good eye contact, increasing the intimacy of the pose. He can help support your leg that is wrapped around him by anchoring it to his hip.

Position 44 – The Cyclist

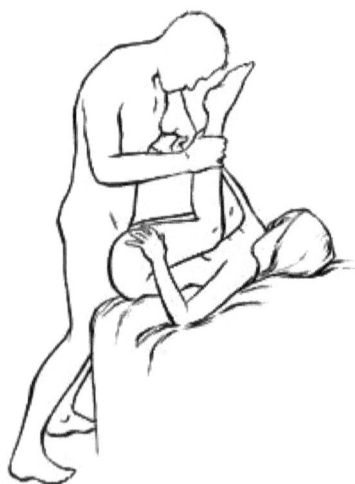

You'll enjoy pedaling your way to ecstasy in this position. Start by lying on the very edge of the bed and pulling your legs up. Your partner will stand next to the bed and enter you. Depending on his height, this could be a very different angle than when you are lying flat on the bed. He will grasp your ankles, and as he thrusts, you move your legs like you're pedaling a bicycle. The motion will move him inside you, creating different sensations. The Cyclist allows for very deep penetration. You'll need a good bit of flexibility through your hips, knees, and lower back to complete the motion. Your partner gets a great view of himself sliding into you while you are treated to a view of his face and body as he thrusts inside you.

Position 45 - Pile Driver

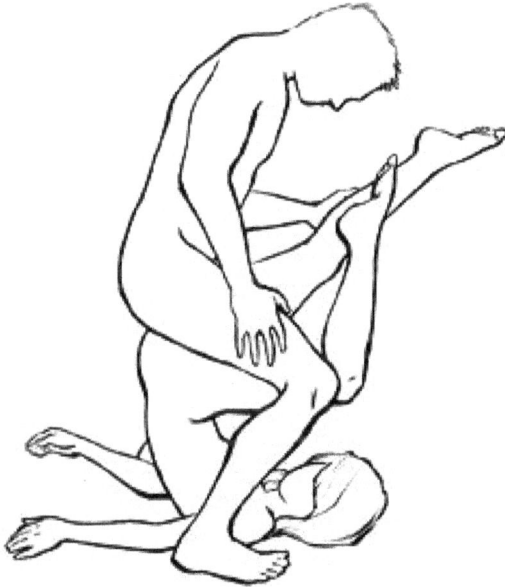

This position requires good flexibility and excellent core strength on your part and good lower body strength from your partner. There is also a risk of putting too much strain on your back and shoulders if he is unable to fully bear his own weight. It is important if either one of you is getting tired to switch out to a new position. This position can be a little tricky to get into and is easier on a firm surface.

You'll begin by raising your legs up and over your head, keeping your shoulders on the ground. Your partner will squat over you and slide himself straight down into your vagina. He can help you maintain your position by holding your legs. Bending a leg, like in the illustration, helps maintain balance, offers better access for him, and lessens the strain on your back. As he rises from his squat, he can withdraw completely and then enter you again with his next motion. It is up to you to communicate if he can go deeper, or if he is putting too much pressure on your back.

Position 46 - The Plow

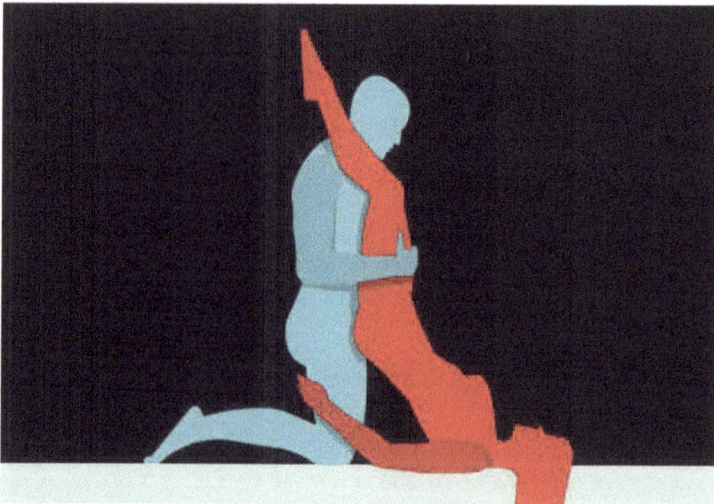

In this position, you'll have your legs supported on his torso and shoulders. You'll want your shoulders to be fairly close to his knees and should be able to grab the backside of his legs. Keep your shoulder blades firmly on the floor or bed. Put your legs up one at a time, and let him help support and balance you. The angle of entry puts a lot of pressure against the top wall of your vagina, stimulating your G-spot. This might look awkward, but if you're able to achieve good penetration, the added pleasure will be well worth the effort. Height differences can prove challenging, and it does require good flexibility and core strength on your part. If you're both comfortable in the pose, widen your legs and let him stimulate your clit while he thrusts to really drive you crazy.

If you're not able to sustain the position on your shoulders, pile up pillows under your hips. Your goal is for him to enter you with an upward stroke. Anything that can put your hips just a bit higher than his will work. Get creative so you don't miss out on the intense sensations offered by this position.

Position 47 - Cowgirl Reversed

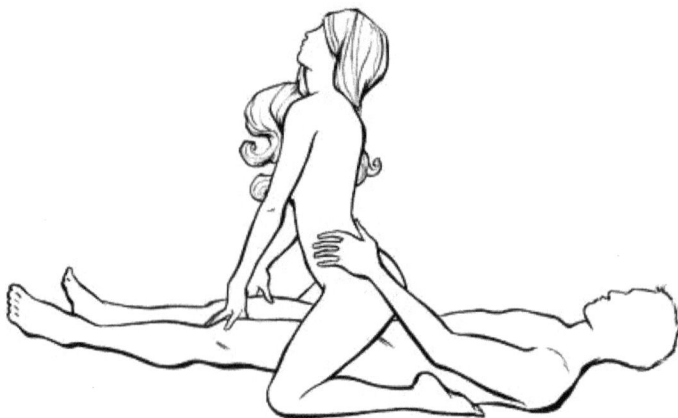

This position turns the woman around from the Classic Cowgirl. This simple position adjustment changes many things. Obviously, it is a different view for your partner, and most men love to have such a great view of their partner's backside. The angle of entry is different, and by adjusting the angle of your upper body, you can adjust it and the depth of penetration. Climb on board for a whole new ride!

Position 48 – Twisted Cowgirl

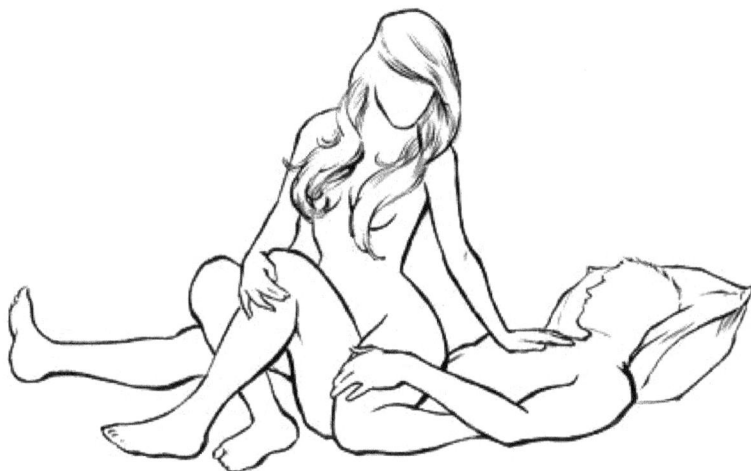

This position offers double pleasure for you. To settle into the position, have your partner lay back and bend one knee. Straddle his bent leg and lower yourself onto him. You can use his leg as leverage as you rock up and down. Press your vulva tightly against his leg to increase stimulation and pleasure. He gets an extra treat of watching your backside, and if he props himself up with a pillow or on his arms, he can see himself as he enters you. To spice it up, play with his balls or lightly trace his perineum.

Position 49 – Wheelbarrow

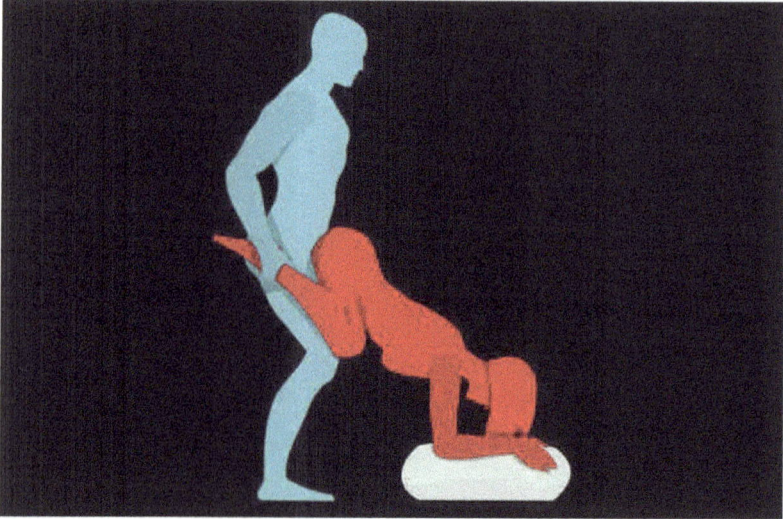

This one takes us back to childhood when we had wheelbarrow races. Just like then, you have to have the upper body strength to support yourself and the core strength to support your back and maintain your position. To get into this position, you bend at the waist and transfer your body weight to your arms. Bracing yourself on your forearms like pictured above is far more stable than arms straight. Lift one leg, bent at the knee, and your partner will anchor it to his hip. Lift the other knee, and once he has you firmly against his hips, let your hips relax toward him while he steps into you. This standing position can be a lot of fun, but if it is too much for your upper body, you can do it seated as well. Your partner sits on the edge of the bed, and you straddle him, reminiscent of Reverse Cowgirl. Spread your legs wider, and lower your upper body toward the floor, and bear part of your weight by putting your hands down.

Position 50 - Classic Doggie Style

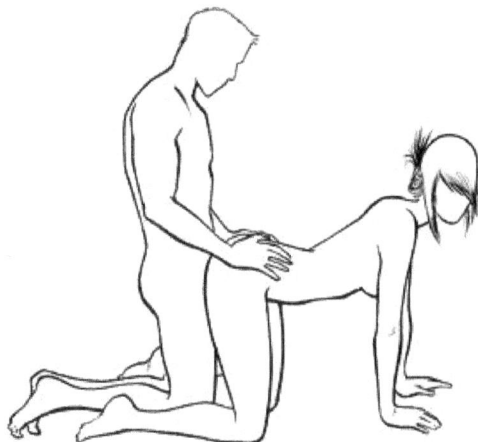

This is another classic position and is a favorite of many men (and women too!). It allows for deep penetration, offers an extremely exciting view for the man, and can hit new angles for you. To assume this position, you'll get on all fours and spread your knees wide. Your partner will kneel behind you and enter your vagina from behind. Height differences can make this one a challenge. Spread your knees wider if your hips are higher than your partner's. You can rock back to meet your partner as he thrusts to increase intensity. There are lots of ways to add excitement to this position. He can reach forward and play with your breasts. You can reach back and play with your clit, or cup his balls in your hand. Spanking often accompanies this position, but make sure that you're both on board with it, and keep it to a level that is pleasurable for both partners. The back is an erogenous zone that is often ignored but is fully exposed in this posture. Your partner can kiss and caress your back and shoulders to find all of your favorite spots.

Rear-facing positions often generate a lot of friction. This can lead to increased pleasure, but also can lead to dryness and micro tears of the vaginal walls or along the shaft of the penis. These tears can cause discomfort, or become infected. The use of lubrication in rear-facing positions is recommended at the first sign of increased friction. There are lots of lubrication options, and you should experiment with different ones to find the best one for you and your partner. Just make sure that they are water-soluble and safe to use internally.

Position 51 - Elevated Doggie

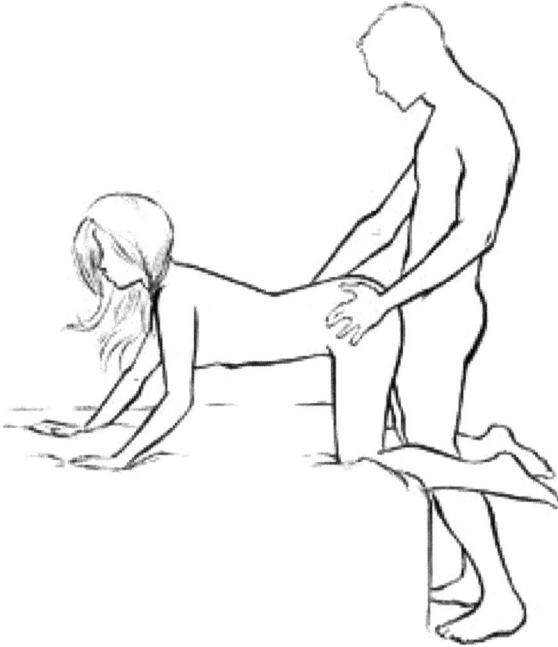

For this position, your partner will stand at the edge of the bed while you are on all fours with your knees spread wide. This is a good way to adjust for height differences. Deep penetration and good support for you are benefits of this position. As with most rear-facing positions, intimacy is not at its height due to the lack of eye contact, inability to kiss and touch, and minimal skin-to-skin contact. You'll need a bit of upper body strength especially if your partner uses powerful thrusts.

Position 52- Steamroller

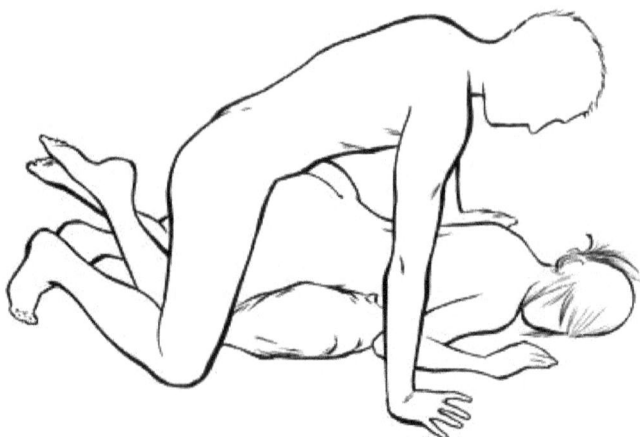

This version of doggie style lets you lay flat on stomach. It is best if you have several pillows under your hips to raise you up off of the bed. Your partner kneels, straddling your legs and enters you from behind just like in doggie style. This angle will be more downward with this position. Since you do not have to bear your weight, it is a good option if you have knee or upper body issues. It can be a bit strenuous on your lower back if you are not in a good position or well-supported under your hips. You also aren't easily able to stimulate your clitoris or see much of anything. If you like your partner in a dominant position, this is a good one to try. Also, you can vary the position by your partner kneeling between your legs.

Position 53 - Monkey See

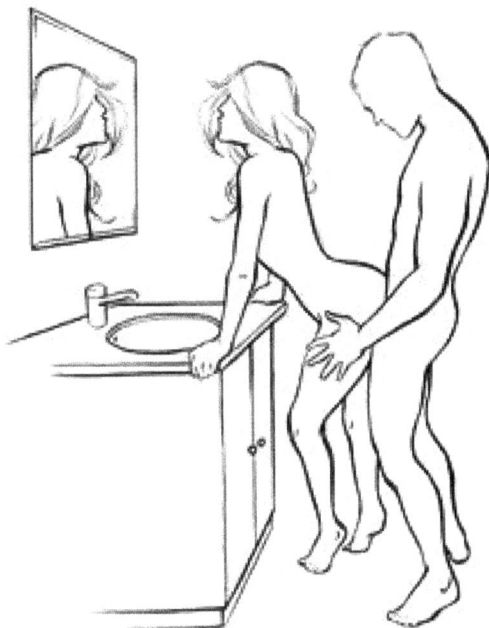

This is the quintessential position for a quickie in the bathroom at a party. It can be done in tight quarters and with minimal removal of clothing if needed. You'll stand braced against the vanity, leaning slightly forward. Your partner will enter you from behind and can use your hips for leverage as he thrusts. While this position isn't reserved strictly for the bathroom, having a mirror to watch the action is an added bonus. Height discrepancies can be tricky, but can be overcome by standing on a small step or a stack of towels.

Position 54 - Spoons in a Drawer

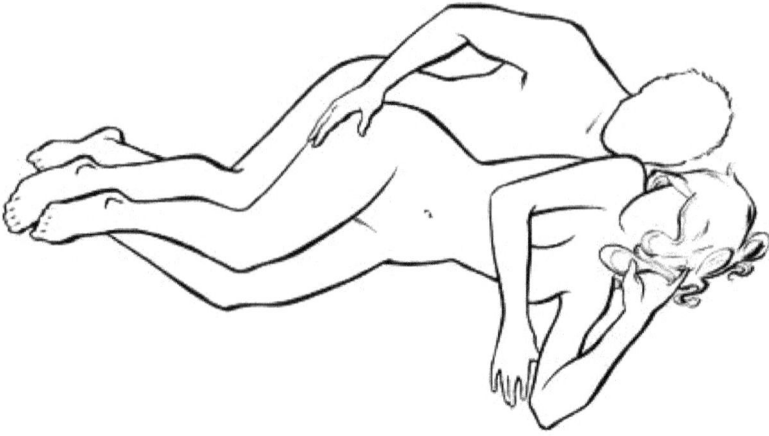

Spooning in bed is relaxing, comforting, and incredibly intimate. Sex in this position is gentle and has shallow penetration. Simply open your legs and allow your partner to slide inside you from behind. To increase depth and contact, drape your top leg back over his hip if you have the flexibility. This position offers full body, skin-to-skin contact and lots of touching and fondling. It is a great position for late pregnancy as well.

Position 55 - Pendulum

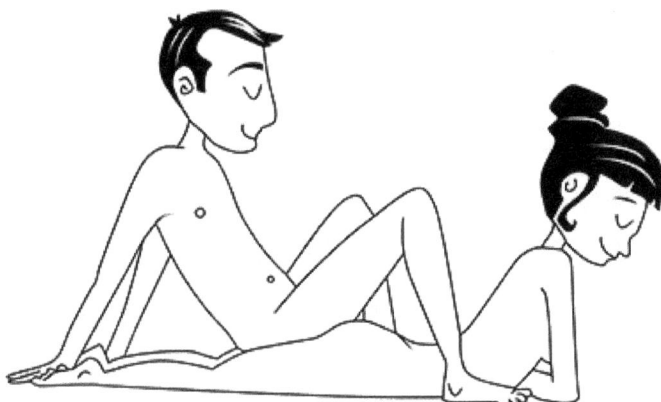

This position is an adventure into new and varying angles of penetration. To begin, you'll lie on your stomach, propped up on your forearms. Spread your legs, and your partner will enter you by sliding down from your butt and leaning back slightly to allow entry. He will move in and out of you by supporting his weight on his arms and legs and swinging his hips like a pendulum. You can keep your legs spread or bring your thighs together to increase the tightness of the penetration. He will need a bit of strength and stamina to keep this one up for long. He can change the level of his hips to adjust the angle and hit different spots of pleasure for you. This is not a highly intimate posture. You are not able to stimulate your clitoris, but he gets a good view of his penis entering you and your backside.

Position 56 - Couch Potato

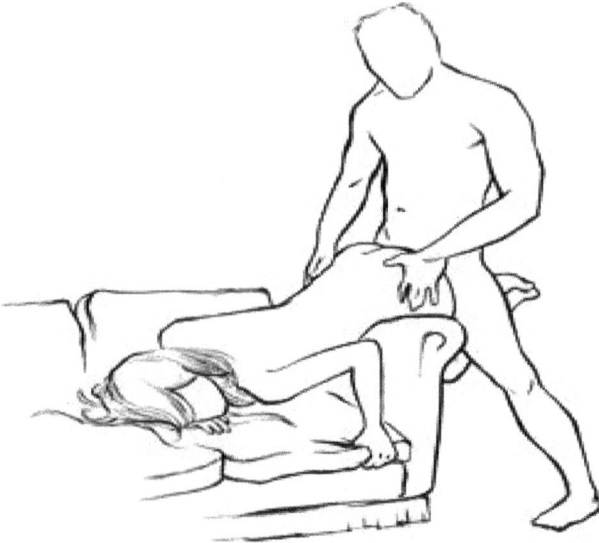

You'll need a couch or a loveseat for this position, but you won't be vegging out and channel surfing. Fold yourself over the arm of the couch, letting your weight rest across your pelvis, and brace yourself on your upper arms. Your partner straddles your legs and enters you. Pick your feet up from the floor if you're able to allow for more freedom of movement. The key difference here is your legs are together between your partner's legs. This allows for a nice, tight hold on him as he thrusts his hips.

Position 57 - Fallen Angel

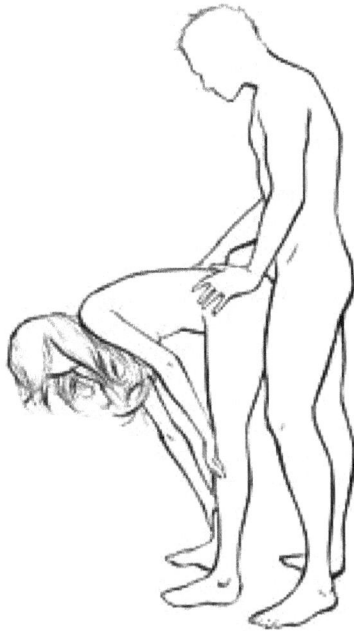

This position can be a great alternative to Doggie Style for people who have bad knees. Standing with legs straight and spread wide, bend at the waist. Your partner will enter you from behind and hold onto your hips. You'll need to trust your partner to hold your hips tightly especially if he is thrusting with a lot of force. To increase intensity, try to rock back to meet him or arch your back for a different angle. If you are secure enough in the position, you can massage your clit or fondle his testicles for added stimulation. You can also put your hands on the floor. Experiment with your hand placement by moving them closer or further away from your feet. This will vary the amount of weight you're bearing on your upper body. You can bend your knees if you need to. If you don't have enough flexibility to reach the floor, or it is hard on your back, try using a chair to brace your arms. This will help with your balance as well.

Position 58 - Stairway to Pleasure

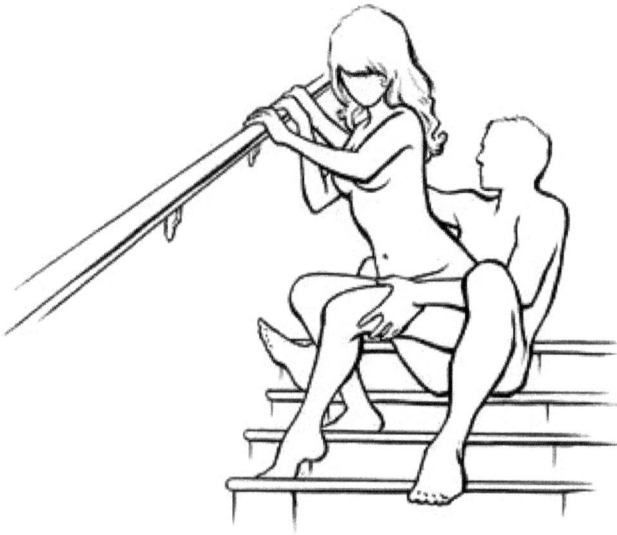

Just can't make it to the bedroom? No worries, using the stairs offers an opportunity for a new position. Your partner sits on a stair, and you'll lower yourself back onto his lap. Your feet will be a stair or two lower than the one he is sitting on. You can be inside his spread legs or straddle his legs if they are together. You get the added support of the rail to grab hold of and use for leverage as you move. If you need a break, lean back against him, and let him explore your body while he nibbles on your neck and shoulders. Taking sex out of the bedroom is a great way to add variety and excitement!

Position 59 - Massage Me

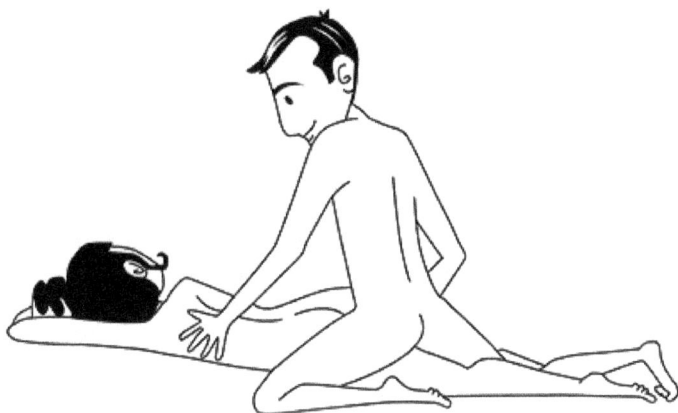

Are you ready to be pampered? This position is all about relaxation. It is a perfect culmination or a slight detour during a massage. As you lay on your stomach, draw one of your legs up and out to the side. You'll naturally be leaning a bit to the side, bringing your hips up nicely for your partner to slide into you. He will straddle your straight leg, entering you from behind. He can continue his massages while he slowly slides in and out, increasing your pleasure. Break out the massage oil, and get ready to think about backrubs in a whole different light!

Position 60 - Hot Seat

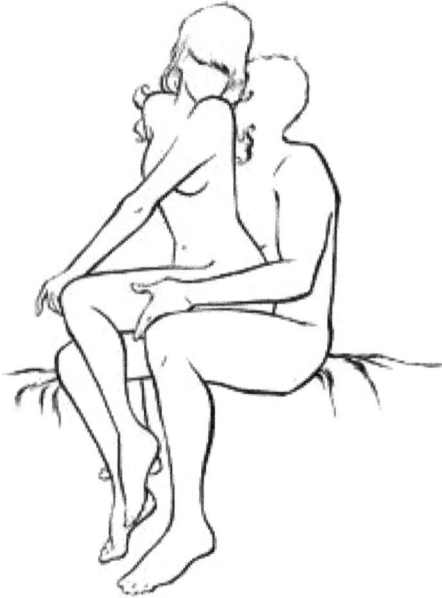

This rear facing position allows for more intimacy than typically found in these positions. Your partner sits on the edge of the bed, usually with one leg on the floor and the other on the bed, either out straight or bent at the knee based on his comfort. He can also have both feet on the floor. You'll lower yourself onto him and sit in his lap with your legs together. You can lean to the side as you rock your hips for a different angle, or just raise and lower yourself like you are pushing up from or lowering into a chair. You can also spread your legs wide, draping one outside of his leg that is touching the floor. This will let him or you reach your clit. Lean back against him to open your upper body for him to touch.

Position 61 - Pleasurable Crab

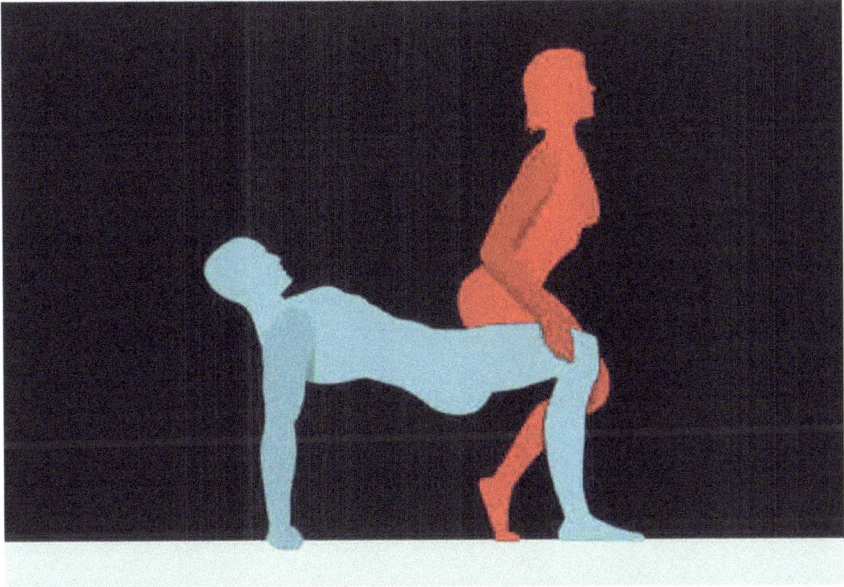

For this position, your partner assumes the crab or reverse tabletop position. This will take a fair amount of strength to hold for long. Support under his hips like an exercise ball or an ottoman will help him hold it longer. This position offers you great control. You'll position yourself between his legs and lower yourself onto his penis. From there, you're the driver. You control the depth and rate of penetration. You can widen your stance and reach down to rub your clit or play with his balls. Brace yourself on his thighs, and go for it! Do be careful as you lower your weight that he is aligned properly. This one can result in penile injury if you come down at the wrong angle with a lot of force. An ER visit will definitely put a damper on the experience!

Position 62 - Roman Candle

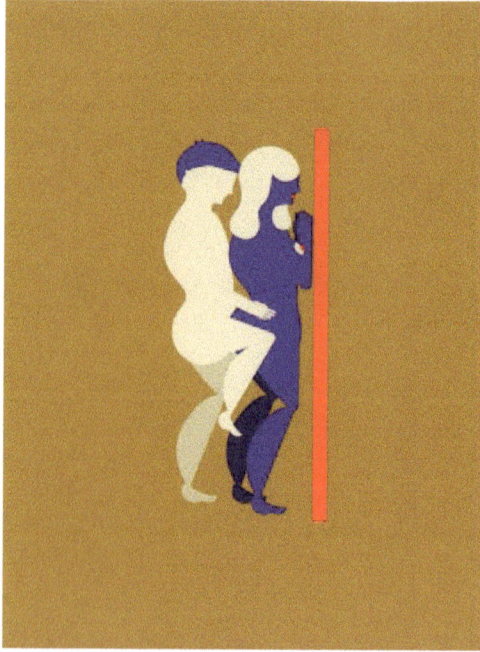

This position is as straightforward as it gets, but can still be incredibly erotic. Perfect for tight spaces, like in the shower, you and your partner both are upright. Widen your stance a bit to allow him entry. A chair or small step for you or him to prop your foot up can also help with alignment. A wall for support is good and adds a layer of eroticism as he pushes you against it. This is another very dominant position. You can feel his body pressing all along your back, and there can be a sense of captivity if he is caging you in with his body. If that makes you uncomfortable, let him be the one against the wall. Differences in height again can make this one tricky, but it doesn't require an extreme amount of athleticism or flexibility from either one of you.

Position 63 - Wilted Flower

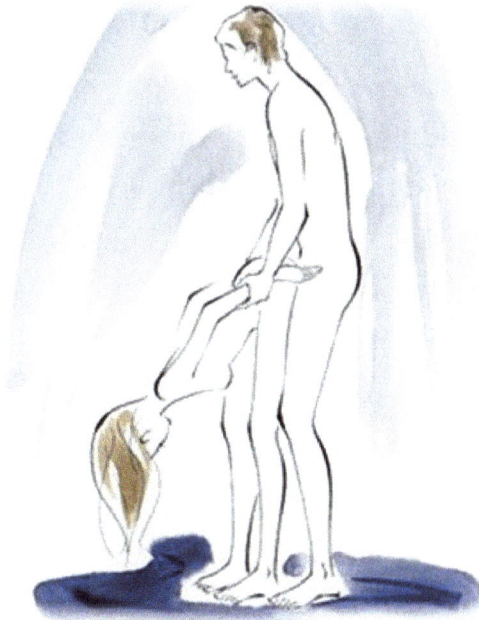

This position can be highly erotic and exciting. You bend at the waist and open your stance wide. Your partner will grasp your wrists or forearms as he enters you. You'll need to have flexibility in your shoulders for this and let him know if he pulls too much. The arm position allows for good leverage, and your wide stance allows for deep penetration.

Anal Sex

Anal sex is seen by many as taboo or risqué. However, it has become more and more mainstream in the last couple of decades. Still, a lot of people shy away from it, particularly women. They think that it is unsanitary, gross or could never be pleasurable. However, the anus has tons of nerve endings, and can be highly erogenous when properly stimulated. Anal sex is something that should be approached with deliberation and good communication between you and your partner. It should be pleasurable and should never cause pain or bleeding. If it does, then something isn't right, and you need to stop until you figure it out.

Here are a few general words of advice before we get into the actual positions:

- To decrease the "gross" factor, be shower fresh, and you can consider a douche or enema before sex. This will free your mind from any worry about smell or fecal matter.
- You can use a condom or a glove, if fingering, to help your partner overcome any squeamishness he might have.
- Go slowly at first. Start gently with fingers and shallow penetration before building up to penetration with his penis or toys.

- Speaking of toys, these are a great way to achieve the anal stimulation that you are craving if your partner isn't into anal sex. There are a variety of toys in all shapes and sizes with different bells and whistles. Find something that you and your partner are comfortable with if you choose to bring a toy into the bedroom.
- Lubrication is a must. The anus doesn't self-lubricate like the vagina. You'll need to find a water-soluble lube that is safe for sex and internal use. There are many on the market to choose from. When it comes to anal sex, the more the better!
- Relaxation is the key for enjoyment. Lots of foreplay can build your excitement. Tell your partner if something isn't right, and only take this step with a partner who you trust and are comfortable with (particularly if anal is new to you!).

Anal foreplay- Before deep penetration, the anal sphincter needs time to loosen and get used to the size it is expected to accommodate. This is a crucial aspect if you are going to enjoy anal sex. While this is written from the viewpoint of the woman, many men enjoy anal stimulation and penetration as well.

Begin with rimming. This is basically a massage just inside and around the anus. It increases blood flow to the area and loosens the muscles of the sphincter. Coupled with clitoral stimulation or kissing, it is often extremely pleasurable to the point of orgasm in some cases. Don't forget the lube!

Once things are loosened up, your partner can slide a finger slowly deeper into the anus, again with plenty of lube. If you start to get tense, take some deep breaths and try to relax. Tell your partner to go slowly, and consider rolling your nipples, or stroking your clitoris to help move your focus elsewhere. Your partner can gradually add another finger or two as you are ready.

If you are enjoying the sensations and are ready for it, try some of these positions with full anal penetration from your partner.

Position 64 - Parting the Rose

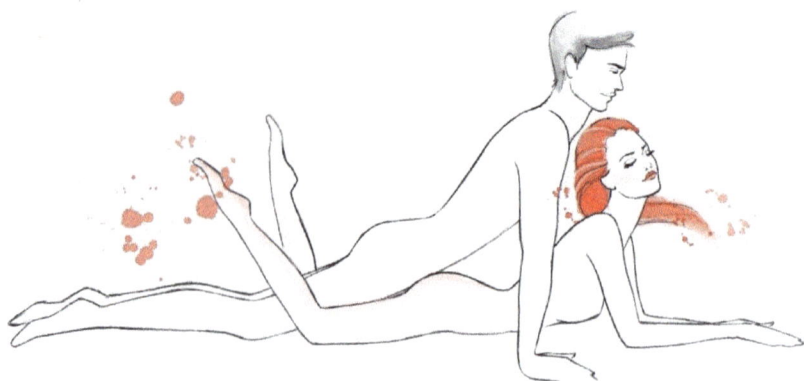

This position is a good beginner's position. Penetration can be controlled easily by your partner and can gradually get deeper as you get more comfortable. You will lie on your stomach and spread your legs. Your partner will kneel between your legs and enter you from a higher angle than if he were entering your vagina. You can be propped up on your elbows or resting your head on a pillow. Another variation that might be more comfortable if being on your stomach strains your back is to put a pillow or two under your hips.

Position 65 - Sidewinder

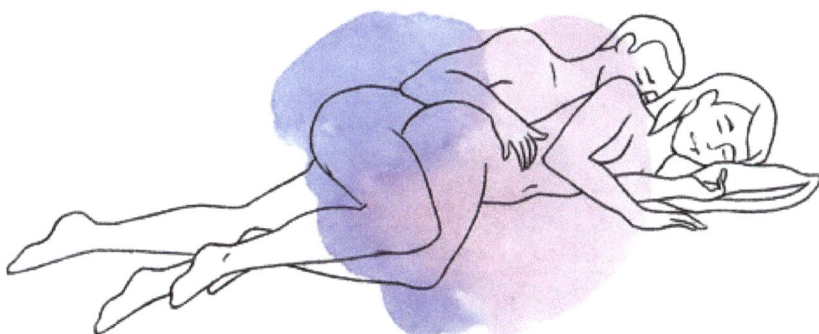

This pose is a very intimate position. Your partner can cuddle and cradle you as he enters you. The motions are typically gentler since forceful thrusting can be difficult in this position. Lying on your side with your partner behind you, pull your top leg up, bending at the knee. Your partner's leg will travel with yours as he enters you and pulls your hips tightly into his. Varying his position behind you, closer to your head or your feet, will alter the angle and sensations for you. This position also allows you or him to stimulate your clitoris for added pleasure.

Position 66 - Table for Two

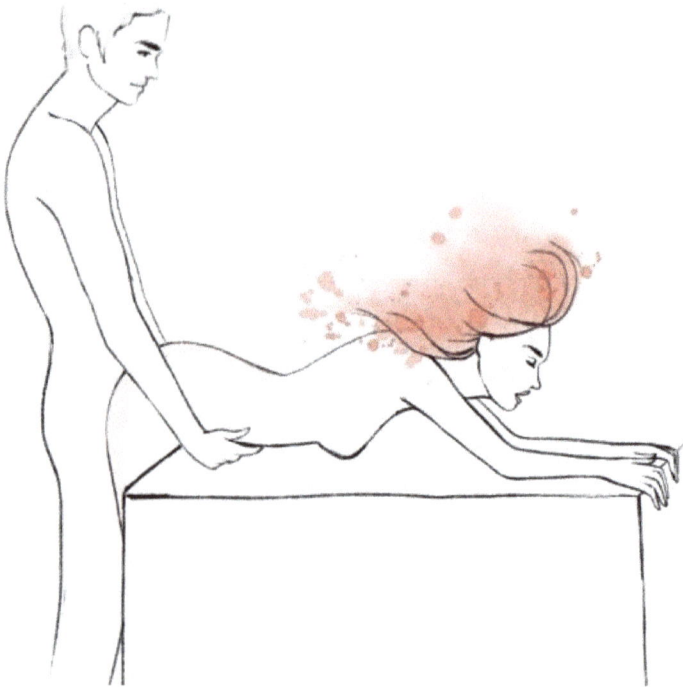

This standing variation requires you to have something to bend over to support your upper body. You can use a table, a counter, or the bed. Your stance can be closed or wide open, whatever works best for you. Your partner will stand behind you and slide himself into you. This is a great position for him to take his time and stimulate you with his fingers or the tip of his penis before diving in for deep penetration.

Position 67 - Good Dog

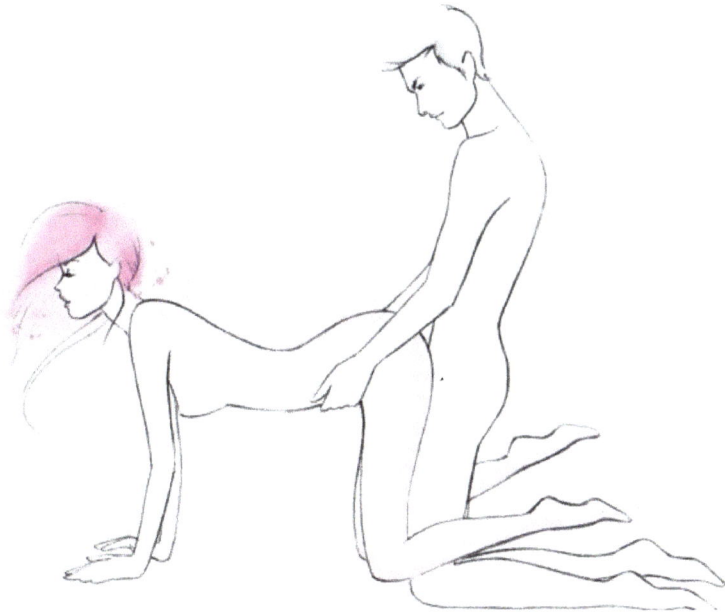

Just like in the vaginal position of Doggie Style, you are on all fours, and your partner is behind you. This posture requires that you can support your weight on your hands and knees. Spread your knees wide to allow him the best access. With a wide stance, you are open for him to stroke your clit, and use his fingers in all sorts of clever ways before entering your rosebud. This position can provide very deep penetration, and is a favorite among men for the great view of him sliding into you. Try changing from vaginal to anal sex in this position for more variety.

Position 68 - Have a Seat

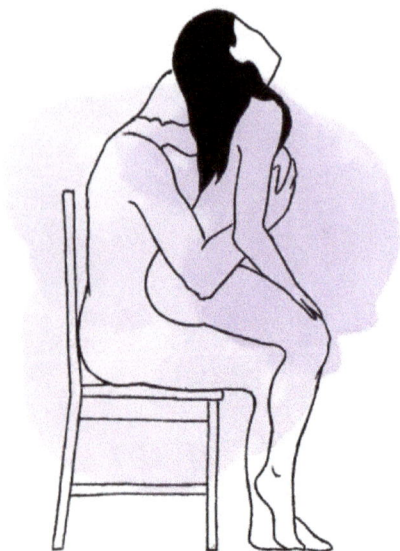

This seated position offers a deep penetration while still allowing you to maintain control of the movement and tempo. Your partner will sit on a chair or the edge of the bed. You will turn away from him before sitting back and allowing him to enter you. Your legs can be spread wide and straddling his or can be closed and in between his. Try it both ways to decide what feels best. As you settle back on to him, go slowly and allow him to guide the alignment. You might have to spread your cheeks a bit to help him aim correctly. Once you're settled, you're in a great position to lean back against him and let his hands explore you.

Position 69 - The Flower

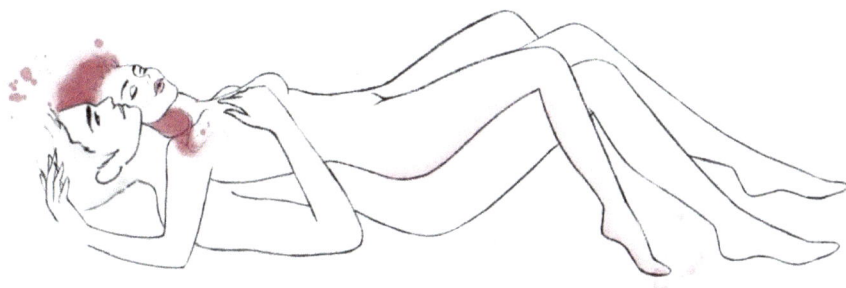

This position is one of the most intimate of all anal positions. Your body is draped over your partner. The complete skin-to-skin contact coupled with the opportunity for kissing, touching, and talking contribute to its intimacy. To achieve this position, straddle your partner's hips facing his feet. It might help if he is propped up or sitting up. Slide back onto him, and then lay back together. He can rock his hips, or you can bend your knees, and raise and lower your hips.

Before we finish please see my other book:

Tantric Sex: A Tantric Massage & Positions Guide to Unleash Your Inner Shiva & Shakti with Pictures by me, Olivia Love

Final Thoughts

You now have 69 fresh ideas to add variety to your sex life. Keep an open mind about the positions. Don't look at them, and immediately decide you can't do it. You are braver and stronger than you know. Maybe you can't keep a position for a long time, but that doesn't mean that for the short time you can do it, it won't feel amazing. One of the best things about sex, like any physical activity, is that it gets better with practice. Sounds like a great excuse to have more sex!

Reading and thinking about these positions are just the first steps. Sometimes, the next step is the biggest hurdle. Talking with your partner can be difficult at first, but once you open the dialogue, it gets easier and easier to talk about trying new things. Use the images in the book if you find it hard to describe what you want. The key is to have open and honest communication about what each of you wants in your sex life.

You've taken a bold step in educating yourself in ways to improve this vital part of your well-being. Don't let your journey stop with these pages. Continue to seek new ways to keep your sex life fun and fresh!

9 781838 432201